Praise for *The Smart Mediterranean Diet Cookbook*

"It's one thing to understand the science behind nutrients and brain health, but it's another thing to prepare meals based on that knowledge. Thankfully, *The Smart Mediterranean Diet Cookbook* gives you all the tools you need to make this way of eating quick, easy, and delicious! Each recipe uses ingredients that contain key nutrients necessary for optimizing cognition and mood, as well as important anti-inflammatory compounds that are vital for not only brain health, but overall health and disease prevention. To top it off, the recipes are simple and family friendly. This cookbook is a winner all the way around!"

CAROLYN WILLIAMS, PHD, RD, anti-inflammatory expert, author of *Meals That Heal* and *Meals That Heal One Pot*, cohost of *The Happy Eating Podcast*, and James Beard Journalism Award winner

"As research continues to show that what's good for heart health is also good for brain health, *The Smart Mediterranean Diet Cookbook* shares tasty tips, tools, and recipes to bring the Mediterranean flavors and health benefits to your own table. Deanna and Serena have delivered, once again, on the delicious and nutritious ways we can enjoy our food with health in mind."

MELISSA JOY DOBBINS, MS, RDN, CDCES, award-winning dietitian and diabetes educator, and host of the *Sound Bites* Podcast

"As a practicing neurologist, I understand and observe daily the benefits of a healthy diet on brain function, as well as the consequences of poor nutrition. The Mediterranean diet contains a good balance of the many nutrients that we know are important to maintain this health. I encourage all my patients to maintain this type of good nutrition and this book is a great place to start."

DANIEL MATTSON, MD, neurologist at SSM Health Medical Group in St. Louis

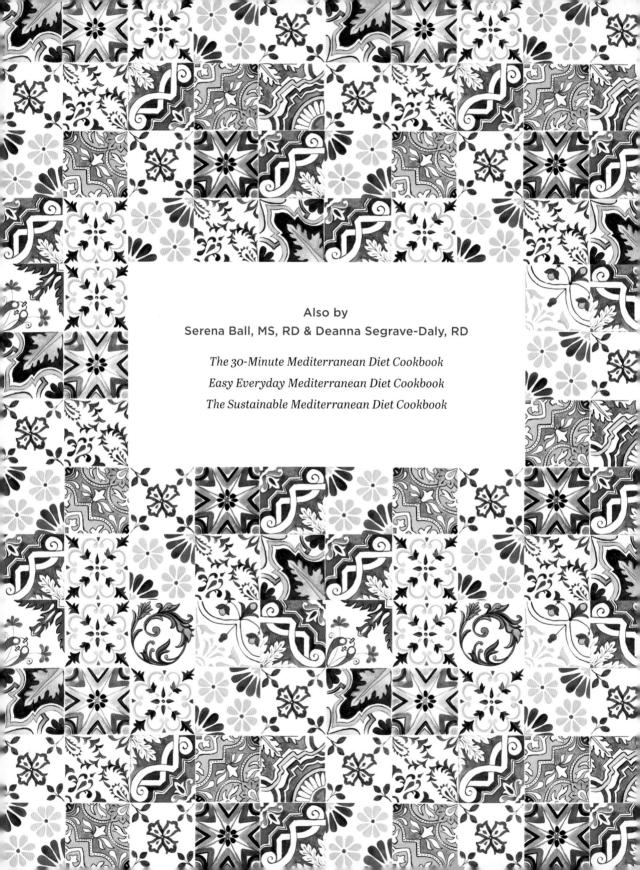

Also by
Serena Ball, MS, RD & Deanna Segrave-Daly, RD

The 30-Minute Mediterranean Diet Cookbook

Easy Everyday Mediterranean Diet Cookbook

The Sustainable Mediterranean Diet Cookbook

The *The* SMART MEDITERRANEAN DIET *Cookbook*

101 Brain-Healthy Recipes to Protect Your Mind and Boost Your Mood

Serena Ball, MS, RD &
Deanna Segrave-Daly, RD

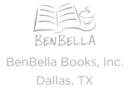

BenBella Books, Inc.
Dallas, TX

Special discounts for bulk sales are available. Please contact bulkorders@benbellabooks.com.

BenBella Books, Inc.
10440 N. Central Expressway
Suite 800
Dallas, TX 75231
benbellabooks.com
Send feedback to
feedback@benbellabooks.com

BenBella is a federally registered trademark.

Printed in China

10 9 8 7 6 5 4 3 2 1

Library of Congress Control Number:
2023033576
ISBN 9781637744505 (trade paperback)
ISBN 9781637744512 (electronic)

Editing by Claire Schulz
Copyediting by Karen Wise
Proofreading by Rebecca Maines
    and Ashley Casteel
Indexing by Debra Bowman
Text design and composition by Tara Long
Cover design by Morgan Carr
Photography by Elise Cellucci
Images on page 15 © Adobe Stock /
    Elena Moiseeva / jul_photolover
Printed by Dream Colour

CONTENTS

INTRODUCTION

What would you think if your doctor wrote you a prescription for a seafood dinner? While it might seem funny to imagine, for many, this is already happening.

Physicians and psychiatrists know that medications can vary in their effectiveness for different individuals, but seafood can help nearly everyone. Its powerful omega-3 fatty acids, selenium, potassium, B vitamins, and other nutrients boost brain health, including (and especially!) mental health—which is why one of the first things many brain health doctors now recommend is to eat seafood often. These and other powerful eating strategies are what make up what we call the "smart" Mediterranean diet lifestyle.

This book will help you seamlessly incorporate this smart lifestyle into your own. The research on the brain benefits of the Mediterranean diet is clear. People who live in Mediterranean regions and more closely follow the Mediterranean diet tend to have a reduced risk for dementia and cognitive decline and fewer psychiatric problems. It also makes sense that this diet, originally linked to heart health, is also good for the brain, as healthy blood vessels that keep blood flowing to the brain reduce the risk of stroke and vascular dementia.

In this book, we've boiled down the large body of neuro-scientific research and used that guidance to create crave-worthy recipes to help keep your brain nourished and sharp for a long life. Start today. Your brain—and the rest of your body!—will benefit, perhaps even immediately. Let this cookbook guide you in learning how simple it can be to cook and eat with your brain in mind!

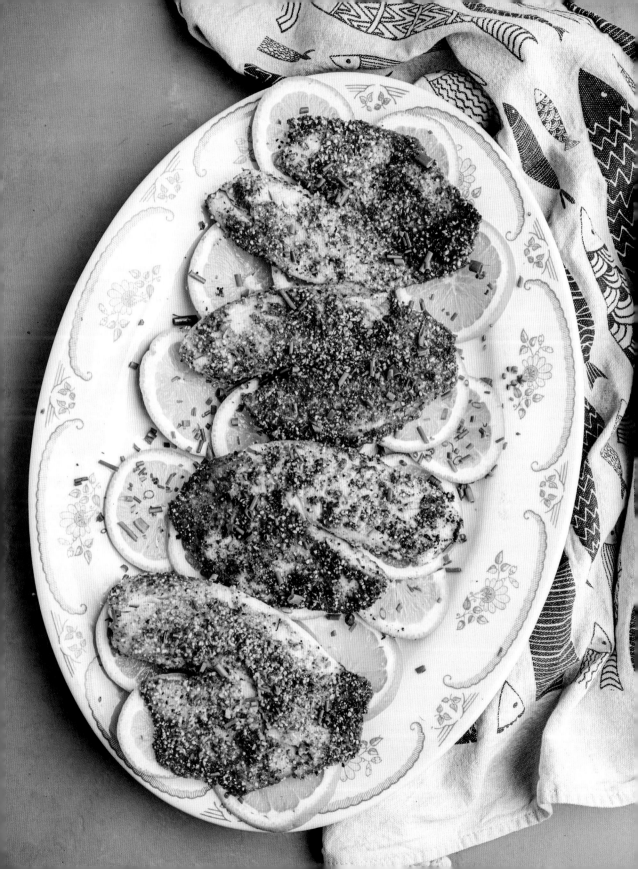

The SMART MEDITERRANEAN WAY

The term "Mediterranean diet" started to be used in the 1960s after nutrition researchers found that working-class communities in Greece and Italy had a low incidence of heart disease, but it has evolved to encompass the similar eating patterns found in the lands surrounding the entire Mediterranean Sea. (And of course, the lifestyle itself goes back centuries!) There are over 20 countries bordering the Mediterranean Sea: Algeria, Tunisia, Libya, Egypt, Palestine, Israel, Lebanon, Syria, Turkey, Cyprus, Greece, Albania, Montenegro, Bosnia and Herzegovina, Croatia, Slovenia, Italy, Malta, France, Monaco, Spain, and Morocco. Specific dishes, spices, and the local ingredients vary greatly from Croatia to Tunisia and from Morocco to Turkey, but all around the coastline, there are similarities in eating patterns that have come to be defined as the Mediterranean (Med) diet.

This eating pattern is primarily based on plants—fresh and local, frozen, or canned. Common ingredients include olive oil as the main fat, whole grains, beans and legumes, nuts and seeds, fruits, vegetables, seafood a few times a week, fermented dairy foods like yogurt and cheese, eggs along with some poultry and meat, and infrequent sweets. Water and wine (for those who drink alcohol) are the main beverages. In many of these countries, we've seen how folks sit around the table to eat in a slow-paced and convivial fashion. Yes, even this style of eating together with others has been shown to improve mental health. Try to eat a congenial meal with family or a coworker (or a former stranger/new friend at a common restaurant table) at least once a day!

Brain health research has exploded in recent years, and scientists and medical professionals are discovering how important the Med diet is for defending and even improving cognitive and mental health.

THE MEDITERRANEAN DIET is bountiful in antioxidant-rich foods, including resveratrol in grapes and wine, lycopene in canned tomatoes, carotenoids in fresh herbs and orange vegetables, capsaicin in spicy peppers, curcuminoids in turmeric, flavones in extra-virgin olive oil, chlorogenic acid in coffee, and many others. Foods containing antioxidants protect the brain from wear and tear, fighting free radicals caused by inflammation that damage brain cells. Antioxidants can also form a layer of protection around healthy brain cells, shielding them from damaging components in the body and in the environment.

EATING MED *for* YOUR BRAIN

Eating according to the Mediterranean diet may help preserve our brain health as we age. When we talk about brain health, most often we're talking about preserving our memory and living free from dementia (defined as a loss of cognitive and physical function that interferes with daily activities). It's estimated that about 1 in 7 people in the US age 71 and older have some form of dementia; among people age 85 and up, the number jumps to half.

Two of the most common causes of dementia are Alzheimer's disease and vascular dementia, or damage to blood vessels that restrict blood flow to the brain. Inflammation in the brain may also play a role. Acute or short-term inflammation can be a good thing; for example, if we cut our finger, the resulting inflammation in the area is temporary and stimulates the immune system to fight infection. However, chronic inflammation, due to age, lack of exercise, and other stressors, is a big risk factor for most chronic diseases, including heart disease, cancer, diabetes, and brain disorders. With Alzheimer's, inflammation in the brain can lead to the buildup of certain proteins, which block the signals between neurons and other communication pathways. Inflammation can also cause the death of brain cells.

However, these changes happen gradually over many years. And, happily, some of them can be slowed or prevented through lifestyle—which is where the Mediterranean diet may help.

Eating according to the Mediterranean diet lifestyle has benefits for memory and cognition. Researchers in a *Journal of the American Geriatrics Society* study observed that Americans in their 60s and 70s who followed a mainly Mediterranean-style diet (eating primarily whole grains, fruits, vegetables, potatoes, legumes, fish, and olive oil) had a 35 percent decrease in risk of cognitive impairment, specifically in long-term and short-term memory and attention.

In a clinical study in the *Journal of the American Medical Association*, researchers conducted a clinical study to determine if people who ate according to the Mediterranean diet (or a lower-fat diet) could decrease cognitive decline. Around 330 people completed the trial, and those eating the Med diet—including increasing their consumption of extra-virgin olive oil or nuts—improved their cognitive function, including scores in memory and executive function (planning, focusing).

Forgetting things as we get older may seem like an unavoidable part of aging, but eating according to the Mediterranean diet may help improve memory. Antioxidants are key (see the box opposite), but so are healthy fats, which are brain food. Beyond fish and olive oil, Med diet foods rich in good fats include walnuts (rich in oleic acid), which can improve memory and brain synapse transmission. Strong memory and brain function are not the only features of a healthy brain. Your mental health matters, too.

MIND *versus* MED

You may have heard of the MIND diet and its link to slowing cognitive decline in healthy older adults. Debuting in 2015, the MIND diet is partially based on the Mediterranean diet; the name stands for Mediterranean-DASH Intervention for Neurodegenerative Delay, where DASH refers to the Dietary Approaches to Stop Hypertension diet. Researchers at Rush University followed over 900 older adults and found that those who most closely followed the MIND diet had a 53 percent lower risk of Alzheimer's, while those who most closely followed the Mediterranean diet reduced their risk by 54 percent.

So, since the Mediterranean diet is part of MIND, what's the difference? There are several. The Mediterranean diet generally includes more fatty fish than does the MIND diet. Research has found a link between eating fish and better mental health (see page 18), and we stand by that. The same is true for eggs, which contain the important nutrients choline and lutein. These nutrients are critical for the brain, but eggs are not encouraged in the MIND diet. The MIND diet does recommend eating beans and lentils every other day (which is a great idea!). But in general, the MIND diet, which limits some fruits and vegetables, is more restrictive than the Mediterranean diet.

The standard Mediterranean diet does not focus on berry consumption as much as the MIND diet does. The research on berries with regard to cognitive health is also strong, so we would encourage you to include lots of berries weekly, fresh or frozen or dried—see page 17 for more. And lastly, the research on the MIND diet is focused on older adults, but we think the benefits of the Mediterranean diet should extend to the whole family!

EATING MED *for* YOUR MOOD

The Mediterranean diet has also been linked to a reduced likelihood of depression in adults. In one 2013 meta-analysis, a higher adherence to the Mediterranean diet was associated with a 30 percent reduced risk for depression. And in a randomized controlled study (the SMILES trial), scientists concluded that a Mediterranean-style diet (including 3 tablespoons of olive oil daily) may be an effective treatment strategy that is accessible to almost everyone—even those unwilling/unable to take medications—for managing major depression.

People with anxiety disorders often have low blood levels of omega-3 fats, so eating more walnuts, flaxseed, and especially fish may help. The Mediterranean diet can even help children, teens, and young adults. Researchers in Australia found that after only 3 weeks of eating a Mediterranean diet, 76 college students prone to depression experienced decreased symptoms of anxiety. In a research review, scientists analyzed 119 papers and found that this diet can be a good prevention strategy, and an effective supportive treatment for anxiety disorders and depression for children and teens. A trial in Spanish children found that better adherence to the Mediterranean diet—marked by fruits, vegetables, pulses more than once weekly, and olive oil consumption—was linked to reduced risk of depression, better physical health, and other quality of life measures.

The diet has also been explored as a treatment for obsessive-compulsive disorder (OCD) and bipolar disorder. Low levels of vitamin B12 and vitamin D, along with high levels of the amino acid homocysteine, may play a role in the development of OCD. In animal studies, probiotics have decreased OCD-like behavior. People suffering from bipolar disorder had improved mood and energy and less irritability with a diet high in omega-3 fats and lower in omega-6 fats than on a control diet. A healthy diet similar to the Mediterranean diet, which is rich in vitamin B12, vitamin D, omega-3 fats, and probiotics could help with these mental disorders.

EATING MED *for* WHOLE-BODY WELLNESS

Of course, the studies have been stacking up for decades, and the Mediterranean lifestyle has been linked to more than brain health. As we mentioned, the Mediterranean diet has long been associated with lower risk of cardiovascular diseases; more recently, it has also been linked to lower rates of arthritis, asthma, cancer, and diabetes. Studies also show that people who follow a Mediterranean lifestyle overall have lower blood pressure, lower blood lipids, and a lower weight. As a result, health professionals for decades have encouraged people to adopt a Mediterranean lifestyle... and now with the positive ties to brain and mental health, there are still more reasons.

Whether a health care professional suggested you follow the Mediterranean diet or you've decided on your own to eat for wellness, we are honored to help. We're registered dietitians, and we'll help you learn more about eating for health and good taste for the whole body, for you and your loved ones.

So, how can you follow the Mediterranean lifestyle and eat with brain and mental health in mind? Luckily, they are basically the same diet! And the rest of this book will help make it easy for you.

EATING SMART

To make it easier to incorporate the Med diet into your daily lifestyle, we came up with a shopping list of smart ingredients. These are the principal recommended foods supported by years of data. They are not a guarantee of brain health, because everyone comes with their own set of unique variables. But this list may help us make the most of our minds and moods so we can share as many memories as possible with loved ones—even memories of meals from this book! After all, sharing meals with friends and family in a spirit of conviviality or friendliness is the Mediterranean way—and we can all raise a glass to that.

Fill Your Smart Cart with:

- Spices, herbs, and seeds
- Extra-virgin olive oil
- Coffee
- Berries (fresh, dried, and frozen)
- Fiber-rich and probiotic foods
- Fish and shellfish

Eat spices, herbs, and seeds daily

Spices, herbs, and seeds lend flavors and textures that make dishes memorable. These ingredients are derived from plants—dried berries, seeds, bark, roots, flowers, and buds. Think of cinnamon bark, whole chiles, dried peppercorn berries, cumin seeds, ginger root, caper flower buds, and cilantro leaves and stems. Plants contain bioactive phytochemicals with antioxidant and anti-inflammatory properties, which help protect the plant from insects and disease and are often still present in the spices we buy at the market. For different reasons, these bioactive components can also protect our health. You may have heard of free radicals, which are unstable molecules that cause damaging chemical reactions in the body. The bioactive components in many spices help stabilize those free radicals and neutralize their damaging effects.

To preserve maximum antioxidant content, flavor, and aroma, we suggest buying some spices—like nutmeg, coriander, caraway, and cumin—in their whole, not ground, form. Smaller, softer seeds, like cumin and caraway, can be used whole in recipes. You can also grind them yourself in a mortar and pestle or an electric spice grinder (peppercorns) or grate with a Microplane (whole nutmeg). When they are ground and then stored, spices and seeds can oxidize (losing antioxidant potential) and lose aroma. That said, the spices we use daily, like cinnamon and cumin, we also buy ground for convenience. (If spices have lost their aroma, simply use more in a recipe.)

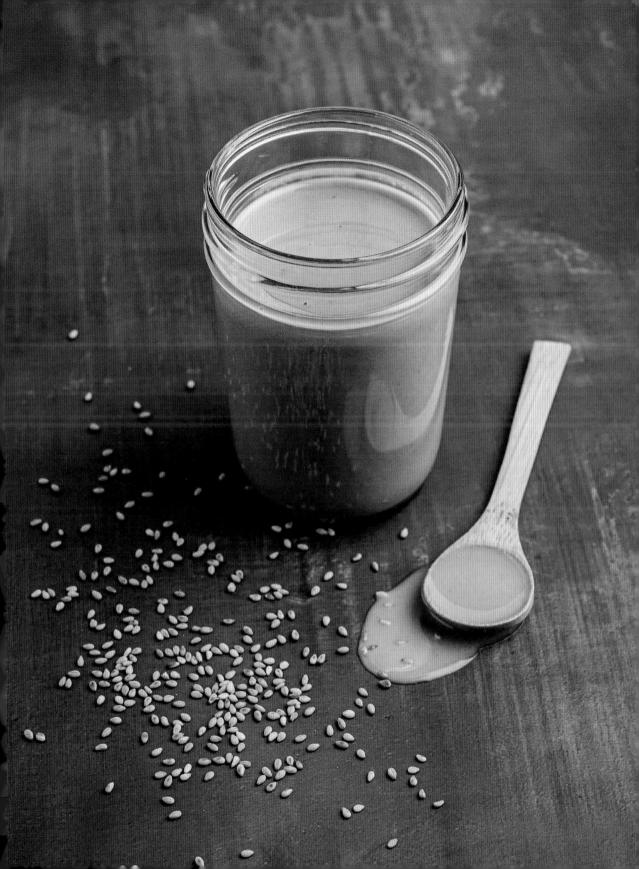

Here's just a sprinkling of the beneficial advantages that these flavorings offer.

Seeds and dried berries. Because seeds contain all the important nutrients and components needed to begin the life of a new plant, they are loaded with fiber, monounsaturated fats, protein, antioxidants, and more. Seeds, especially coriander, cumin, and black pepper, are potent sources of plant antioxidants.

Whole sesame seeds add a slightly sweet nuttiness to many of our recipes, and so does tahini (sesame seed paste), which is popular in Middle Eastern recipes. Researchers conducting animal tests using sesamol, the active ingredient in sesame seeds, found improvements in behavioral memory tests and in some cognitive impairments, potentially from reduced brain plaque.

Black, white, and green peppercorns are actually dried berries. Serena tasted a type of bright red peppercorn berries in Hawaii where they grow on vines (they tasted peppery and fruity!). These red peppercorns dry up, lose their outer hull, and become black peppercorns. Daily use of lots of fresh ground black pepper is an easy way to add a sprinkling of more antioxidants, so add a pepper grinder to your kitchen if you don't have one already.

Roots and bark. Turmeric and ginger are both rhizomes, which are a type of edible plant root. Both have powerful anti-inflammatory components. Turmeric contains curcumin, which can reduce and even correct oxidative stress, the imbalance of free radicals in the body. Some research (both animal and epidemiological studies) on turmeric has shown promise for combating Alzheimer's. Turmeric may even help antidepressants work better, though studies on this have found inconsistent results.

Ginger is also anti-inflammatory and protective for the brain. In animal studies, ginger has been found to help protect against age-related cognitive decline and Alzheimer's-like changes in behavior. A high dose of ginger extract was shown to help middle-aged women do better on tests of reaction time and working memory. Now, our recipes don't contain this high dose of ginger, but the point is that eating a diet rich in many antioxidants means the body is continuously armed with a variety of free radical–fighting weapons.

Cinnamon is made from the inner bark of cinnamon trees and is high in the formidable bioactive cinnamaldehyde. This component may help protect against some of the changes in brain structure that occur with neurodegenerative diseases like Parkinson's and Alzheimer's, although more research is needed.

Chile peppers. Chile peppers are actually fruits, and the capsaicin content of hot chile peppers makes them potent protectors of brain health. Some researchers have even suggested that people at risk for Alzheimer's disease should supplement with capsaicin daily in order to potentially stave off some of the effects of the disease. In animal studies, capsaicin has reduced the blood levels of certain Alzheimer's markers and even reversed cognitive decline. In a clinical study involving people over 40, capsaicin was associated with better cognition and also lower Alzheimer's blood biomarkers. Along with capsaicin, chiles are high in vitamin C, which may help with brain cell protection, growth, and function. Sweet peppers, like bell peppers, are high in vitamin C but have zero capsaicin.

Herbs. Researchers have found that fresh and even dried herbs—including basil, cilantro (often known as coriander outside the US), dill, mint, parsley, rosemary, sage, and tarragon—are rich sources of anti-inflammatory phytochemicals called carotenoids. Basil and cilantro are particularly high in the carotenoids beta-carotene, lutein, and zeaxanthin. These nutrients have been linked to increased cognitive function in young adults (age 18 to 30 years), which shows the importance of a lifetime of healthy eating.

Common Mediterranean dried chiles and chile products

 Urfa (Turkish) — raisin-like fruitiness, almost chocolate-like sweetness, barely hot

 Aleppo (Syrian) — not too spicy, also fruity, hotter than Urfa

 Smoked paprika (Spanish) — smoky with a wide variety of heat levels

 Crushed red pepper (Italian) — hot only

 Shatta (Middle Eastern) — a paste of a variety of chiles, olive oil, salt

 Harissa (Tunisian) — a paste of a variety of chiles, spices, olive oil, salt

Use extra-virgin olive oil daily

Use extra-virgin olive oil as your main fat daily. It's a strong inflammation fighter and is rich in plant phenolic compounds that may counter oxidation in the brain.

Associations between olive oil and cognitive health have been appearing in research journals for the last several decades. In one large randomized controlled study in Spain, researchers found that those following a Mediterranean diet and using 1 liter (about 4 cups) of olive oil per household per week had better cognitive function after about 6 years, and also lower incidence of cognitive impairment or dementia.

It may surprise you that research is also being published about the link between olive oil and mental health.

In Israel, scientists conducted a double-blinded, placebo-controlled study and found that people with symptoms of major depression who consumed about 1½ tablespoons of olive oil a day had significant improvement.

In the "Sun Project," researchers looked at 12,000 middle-aged adults in Spain and found that those who consumed more olive oil had a much lower risk of depression.

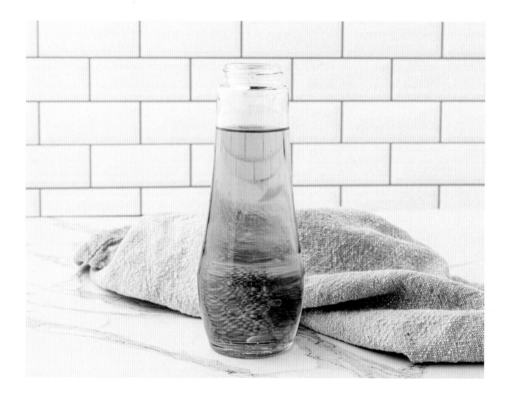

Enjoy berries several times a week

Berries are considered a "gold star" food for brain health. Strawberries, blueberries, blackberries, raspberries, grapes, raisins, and other domestic and wild berries, whether fresh, frozen, or dried, contain a variety of components that may contribute to brain health. Many brain-friendly nutrients like vitamin C, vitamin E, potassium, magnesium, manganese, and fiber are found in berries.

Berries also appear to contain lesser-known components that are associated with brain health. Researchers at Rush University Medical Center found that older people who ate more berries (especially strawberries) over a period of 20 years had fewer of the brain tangles that are hallmarks of Alzheimer's.

Red grapes contain resveratrol, a robust antioxidant that helps protect neurological cells from free radical damage. It can also keep blood vessels healthy, helping to protect against stroke. There is significantly more resveratrol in fresh red/purple grapes and red wine than in green grapes, white wine, and raisins. Drinking a 5-ounce glass of red wine (or grape juice) or eating 1 cup of red table grapes yields around the same amount of resveratrol.

Drink coffee daily

Did you know that coffee beans are actually the seeds of the coffee cherry, the fruit of the coffee tree? After fermentation, the coffee cherries are dried, roasted, and then ground into coffee. Most of the bioactive plant compounds are maintained.

In fact, coffee is the single highest food source of antioxidants in most people's diets. A variety of coffee polyphenols may help target free radicals that can cause brain cell damage. Other antioxidants may help keep brain blood vessels healthy and free from blockage.

In a 10-year study involving over 600 elderly men, those who drank coffee had less cognitive decline than those who did not. Three (small) cups a day seemed to be the sweet spot. Several elements in coffee may be valuable for brain function, including caffeine, which can increase serotonin, the "feel good" chemical that regulates many brain tasks.

Eat fiber and probiotics daily

Fiber keeps you "regular," but it also helps your brain. Many people aren't aware of the strong link between the brain and the gut. (We often say, "I've got a 'gut feeling'" when what we have is a strong thought—and it turns out that saying is truer than we may realize!)

The central nervous system and the intestinal tract are connected in a communication network known as the gut-brain axis. When the gut is healthy, the brain generally is, too. Of course, the opposite can be true. One of the easiest ways to keep the gut healthy is to nourish the good bacteria found there. Dietary fiber keeps the bacteria diverse and plentiful. Most all types of vegetables and fruits contain fiber. But some have a type of fiber that is especially good for feeding good gut bacteria; this is known as prebiotic fiber. These prebiotic foods include onions, garlic, artichokes, leeks, asparagus, apples, barley, and whole-wheat foods. Variety is key to growing diverse and valuable intestinal good bacteria, so mix up your sources: eat lots of legumes, whole grains, and canned, frozen, and fresh fruits and vegetables. (Bonus source: the favorite Mediterranean sweetener, honey, also contains prebiotic carbohydrates.)

Fiber intake has been linked to reduced gut inflammation and stronger memory, and even improved mental health in some population studies, although the research is not always consistent.

Eating foods that contain probiotics—live microorganisms that have a beneficial effect when eaten—has been linked with less depression. In a 2019 study of 26,000 Koreans, those who ate the most fermented dairy foods and fermented vegetables had fewer symptoms of depression than those who didn't eat probiotic foods regularly. Other studies have reported similar associations. The mechanism for this positive effect may be that probiotics help increase the secretion of serotonin and other neurotransmitters. The main sources of probiotics in the Mediterranean diet are yogurt and fermented vegetables.

Probiotics may also help with cognition. A 2021 study of Canadian older adults found that cheese and low-fat dairy intake was associated with better executive functioning (planning, juggling tasks, etc.), and yogurt was further associated with improved memory.

Eat seafood twice a week

In our search for the smartest foods, some of the most compelling research we found suggests that eating fish and some shellfish could be more effective than antidepressants at treating depression in some people.

People who eat fish on a regular basis are 20 percent less likely to have depression than their peers. Dozens of studies over the last two decades have evaluated over 20,000 cases of depression, and the researchers suggest that eating 2 to 3 servings of fish per week can reduce the risk for major depression. The American Psychiatric Association has endorsed fatty acids in fish as an effective part of depression treatment.

In a large study known as the Age-Related Eye Disease Study (AREDS and AREDS2) conducted through the National Eye Institute, researchers found that after 10 years, participants who consumed the greatest amount of fish while also eating a Mediterranean diet had the slowest rate of cognitive decline. Surprisingly, the benefits in this research were independent of whether participants did or did not have the APOE gene, which is a risk factor for Alzheimer's.

Fish benefits the whole family. Pregnant mothers who eat seafood have babies with better outcomes for overall brain and eye wellness. The omega-3 fats found in seafood are crucial molecules that determine the brain's ability to perform. The first 1,000 days of a baby's life (conception to age 2) are the most critical for brain formation, so expectant moms, infants, and toddlers may especially benefit from a few servings of seafood each week. Fish is also linked with children doing better in school, healthy eye development, stronger bones, and even less stress.

One note on mercury: don't worry about it—really! Most fish you'll buy at the grocery store or order at a restaurant is just fine. (According to the FDA, canned tuna, even for pregnant moms and children, is fine to consume, up to 12 ounces weekly.) The only ones to avoid are shark, swordfish, king mackerel, tilefish, and a few lake fish. Fish is also rich in selenium, a nutrient that offsets any ill effects of mercury. Think of selenium as Pac-Man eating up mercury! Low selenium levels in the body have been linked to Alzheimer's disease, brain tumors, and other conditions associated with increased oxidative stress. Ocean fish, which are the most commonly eaten in the US, are among the richest sources of selenium. The bottom line is that seafood provides excellent nutrition, and you don't need to stress about repercussions from mercury exposure.

In general, fish like sardines (probably the best and the most inexpensive), trout, Arctic char, salmon, and many varieties of oysters contain the most omega-3 fatty acids. And these fats are quite literally brain food.

— ❋ —

So there you have it—the top smart ingredients for brain-healthy eating. For more on brain-healthy ingredients, see the chart on pages 22–25. Each of the recipes in this book incorporates at least one of these brain-boosting ingredients.

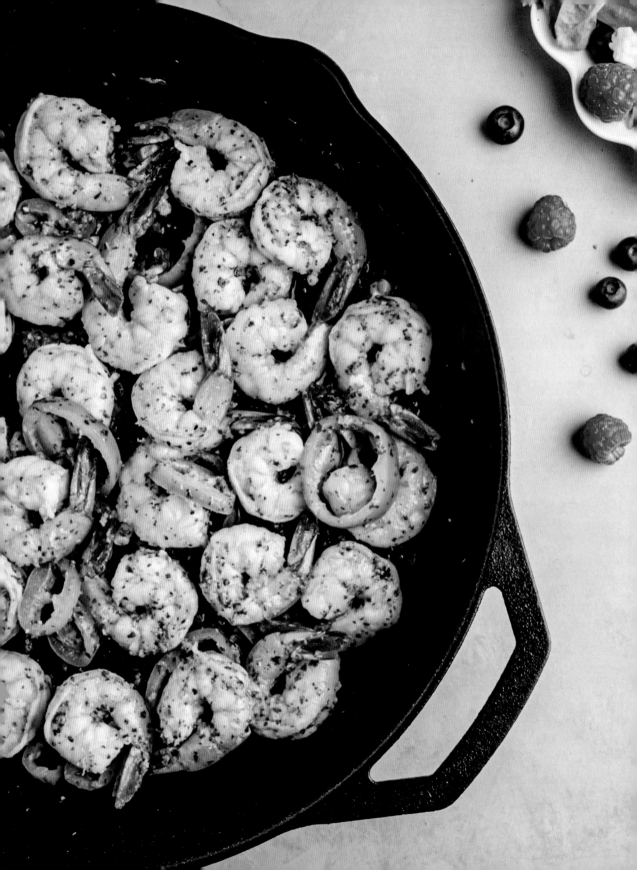

IN THIS BOOK

This is our fourth Mediterranean diet cookbook. Now, we are not experts on authentic cultural cuisines compared to those who are native to Mediterranean regions. However, through our travels and the interviews with acquaintances who grew up in the Mediterranean, we have embraced spices like Aleppo and Urfa peppers on our eggs, and za'atar on our flatbreads. These are recipes we actually feed our families and friends—and have done so for over two decades.

Along the way, we've received emails, DMs, and other messages from hundreds of our readers on how our recipes have helped them and their families get healthier with simple and appealing meals. They are real home cooks who told us what they *really* thought about our recipes and how to make them even better. So we did—everything here has been double- and triple-tested for best flavor and least fuss. And some of those readers have even become recipe testers for this cookbook!

Our readers thank us for using ingredients found in regular grocery stores. And they love our Healthy Kitchen Hacks—tips for ingredient substitutions, kitchen shortcuts, repurposing leftovers, and smart tips that are included with *every single recipe.* Recipes here are flexible for those who want to eat gluten-free, dairy-free, egg-free, nut-free, vegetarian, or vegan. Most of our recipes are packed with plants, but we also include recipes made with shellfish, red meat, and chicken, all rich in B vitamins and zinc (low vitamin-B levels are linked with dementia, and zinc deficiency can lead to brain fog).

Use the meal plans on page 246 to help you get ideas for how to use some of our recipes throughout the week. And while most recipes serve 4 to 6, almost all of them can be halved to feed fewer. (Although having a supply of brain-friendly meals stashed in the freezer is a gift you can give yourself!)

We hope that this cookbook will bring a bit of Mediterranean sunshine to mind whenever you cook from it—and to whomever is joining you at your table!

Cheers to your brain health,

Serena and Deanna

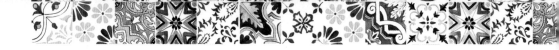

SMART CHART FOODS

Here's the list of foods we recommend to eat more of and the "why?" when it comes to better brain and mental health.

Note: As dietitians, we don't love to single out one nutrient in a food as a silver bullet for health because foods are a full package of nutrients that likely work best together. Case in point: Researchers have found that supplements of omega-3 fats have inconsistently been linked to cognitive and mental health. That said, the body of research on fish and shellfish has more conclusive evidence linking it to positive brain health, probably because in addition to omega-3s, seafood contains a whole host of other brain-friendly nutrients, including selenium, vitamin D, choline, zinc, and B vitamins. Talk about a full package!

Mediterranean Food	Nutrient	Potential Brain Benefit
Hot chiles Crushed red pepper Harissa paste	Capsaicin	Capsaicin is a powerful anti-inflammatory. It may decrease Alzheimer's risk and reduce cognitive decline.
Eggs Shrimp, salmon, tuna, cod Potatoes	Choline	Choline is linked to overall improved brain function, including learning, memory, and mental status, partly because neurotransmitters are partially composed of choline.
Berries	Flavonoids	Flavonoids (there are thousands of types) help reduce the risk of high blood pressure and stroke. They decrease inflammation and potentially the formation of amyloid plaques between neurons in the brain.

Mediterranean Food	Nutrient	Potential Brain Benefit
Citrus fruit Leafy greens (kale, collards, spinach, romaine lettuce) Asparagus Pasta	Folate (a B vitamin)	Low blood folate levels are associated with poor brain function and an increased risk of dementia. Even "normal" but low folate levels are associated with an increased risk of mental impairment in older adults.
Leafy greens Eggs	Lutein	Lutein should be consumed weekly for healthy cognition at every life stage and to help prevent cognitive decline with age. Lutein is 200% more bioavailable in eggs than in vegetables.
Cooked tomatoes (tomato sauce, tomato paste)	Lycopene	Lycopene may help reduce oxidative damage associated with amyloid plaque accumulation in the brain. It may also protect Alzheimer's-affected brain cells from oxidative stress, to help prevent the onset of dementia. Cooking tomatoes breaks down their cell structure to help release more lycopene than is available in raw tomatoes.
Whole grains Dried beans Peanuts, almonds, pistachios, walnuts, sesame seeds, pumpkin seeds Yogurt	Magnesium	Magnesium is critical for relaying communications between the brain and the body. It prevents overstimulation, which can damage brain and nerve cells.
Honey	Oligosaccharides	This prebiotic may help improve the gut-brain axis communication system.
Nuts and seeds (walnuts, almonds, pumpkin seeds, flaxseeds) Kidney beans	Omega-3 fats (plant-based)	The anti-inflammatory properties of omega-3 fats might counteract oxidative processes in the brain that lead to some types of neurodegeneration.

Mediterranean Food	Nutrient	Potential Brain Benefit
Fatty fish (canned sardines, canned tuna, trout, Arctic char, salmon)	Omega-3 fats (animal-based)	Omega-3 fats can improve blood flow to the brain and enhance the synthesis of healthy brain cells, and perhaps decrease the formation of amyloid plaques, a hallmark of Alzheimer's.
Yogurt, labneh, cheese, milk	Potassium and magnesium	These minerals and electrolytes help regulate healthy blood flow to the brain and manage blood pressure to help prevent stroke.
Garlic, onions, scallions, leeks, artichokes, asparagus, apples, barley, whole-wheat foods	Prebiotics	Prebiotics nourish gut bacteria, which helps overall brain health.
Yogurt, labneh, cheese, fermented vegetables	Probiotics	Probiotics can help with mood and decrease risk for anxiety and depression.
Fish and shellfish	Selenium	This powerful antioxidant is highly regulated and conserved in the brain as it's essential for brain function. Selenium also counters any negative effects from consuming mercury. Low selenium levels have been linked to Alzheimer's and many other brain diseases.
Chickpeas Bulgur Potatoes Raisins Milk Beef, lamb Chicken, turkey Seafood	B vitamins (especially vitamins B6 and B12)	Getting enough B-complex vitamins can reduce fatigue and boost mood. Low vitamin-B status is a risk factor for dementia.

Mediterranean Food	Nutrient	Potential Brain Benefit
Citrus fruits Strawberries Cantaloupe Red peppers Broccoli Cabbage Potatoes Tomatoes	Vitamin C	Vitamin C helps reduce free radical damage and inflammation, to preserve brain function.
Mushrooms Milk	Vitamin D	Vitamin D helps the immune system function properly, which directly links to healthy mental health and cognition.
Eggs Leafy greens Whole grains	Vitamin E	This antioxidant has been found to help prevent cognitive delay in elderly people.
Leafy greens Cabbage Brussels sprouts Butter lettuce Parsley	Vitamin K	Vitamin K may slow cognitive impairment and increase learning abilities. It may also help with depression and anxiety.
Oysters, mussels, clams Beef, lamb Chicken	Zinc	Zinc can boost mental performance. It has antioxidant and anti-inflammatory properties, which can help reduce chronic inflammation and mental decline. Low zinc is linked to brain fog.

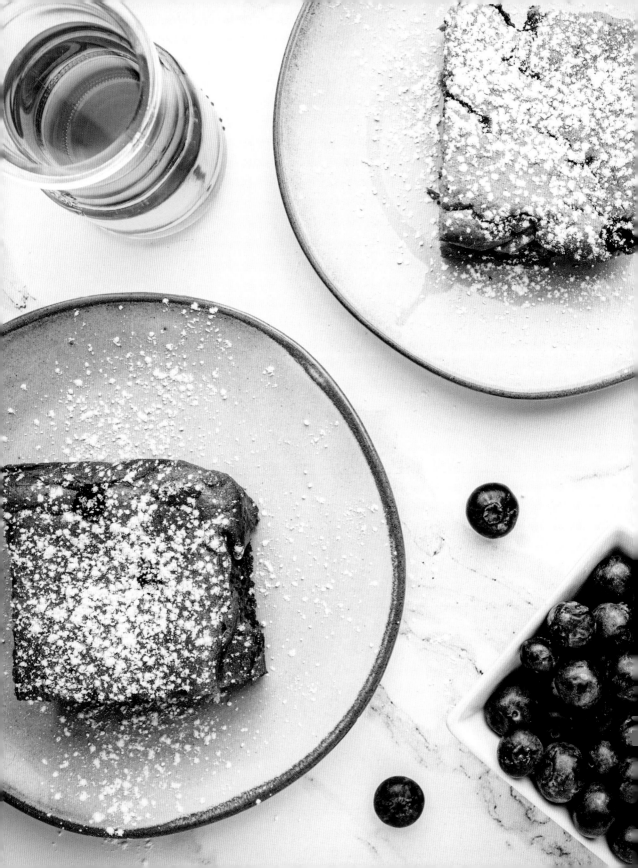

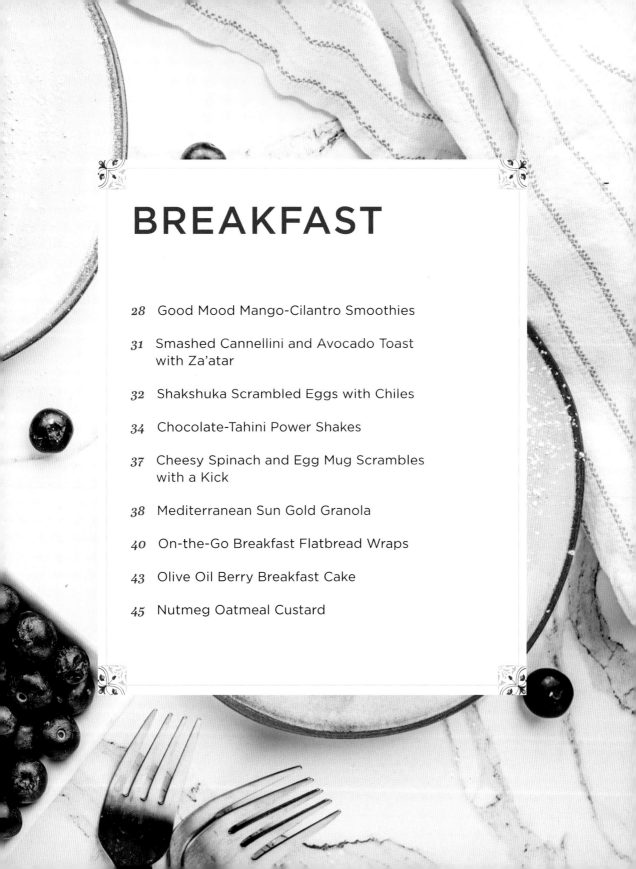

BREAKFAST

Good Mood
MANGO-CILANTRO SMOOTHIES

SERVES 2 Prep time: 5 minutes

1 cup plain kefir

1 cup frozen cubed mango

1 cup fresh cilantro leaves and stems

1 frozen or very ripe banana

⅔ cup orange juice

1 teaspoon honey, plus more for drizzling (optional)

While Deanna has never embraced drinking her greens, she has made this herb-a-licious smoothie time and time again. For its base, she uses kefir, the fermented, probiotic-powered dairy beverage that research suggests may help reduce anxiety and depression. Mixed with a triple dose (mango/orange/cilantro) of vitamin C—a crucial nutrient for brain function and preservation—this bevvy is indeed a smart way to start your day.

Puree the kefir, mango, cilantro, banana, orange juice, and honey in a blender until smooth and the cilantro is pulverized. Divide between two glasses and drizzle the rims with honey, if desired. Serve immediately.

Healthy Kitchen Hack: If you are on "team green smoothie," toss in spinach or kale to your liking. Or use a vanilla-, mango-, or berry-flavored kefir and omit the honey. Or, spice it up with ¼ teaspoon ground ginger per smoothie serving.

PER SERVING: Calories: 202; Total Fat: 2g; Saturated Fat: 1g; Cholesterol: 8mg; Sodium: 69mg; Total Carbohydrates: 43g; Fiber: 3g; Protein: 6g

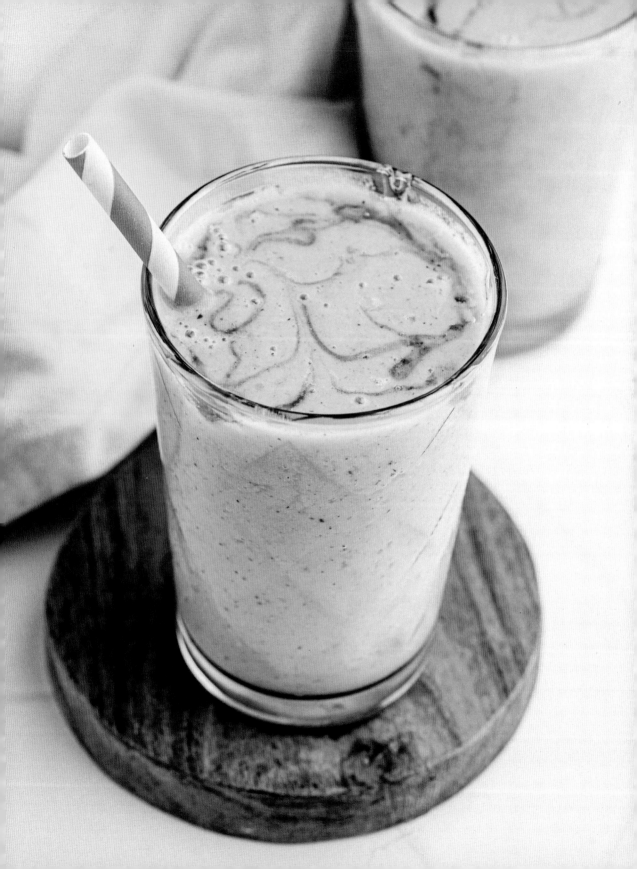

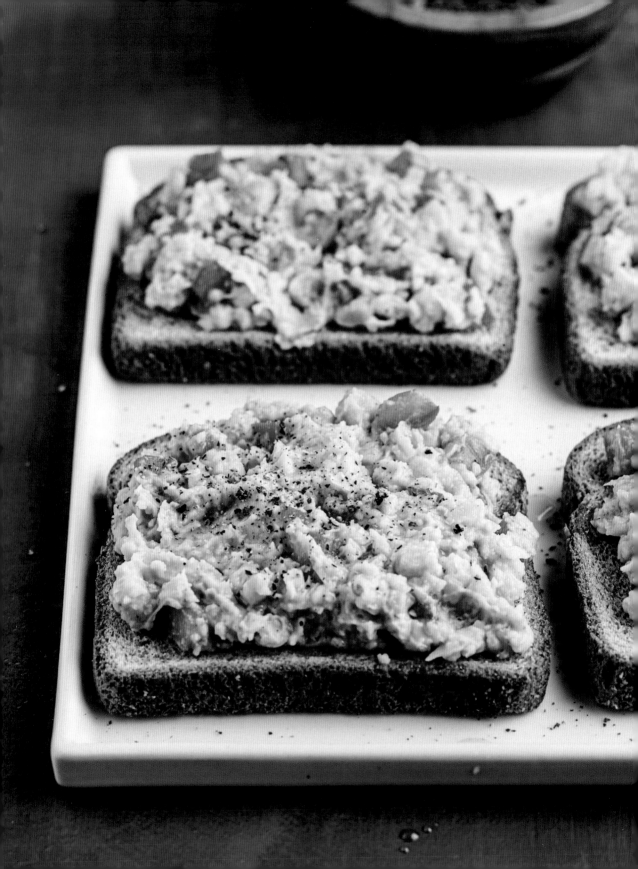

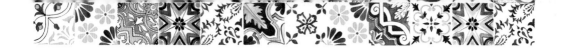

SMASHED CANNELLINI AND AVOCADO TOAST *with Za'atar*

SERVES 4   Prep time: 10 minutes

We have a new appreciation for that trendy toast: our zesty bean version has a stellar combo of brain-boosting nutrients. Not to mention, this energy-sustaining breakfast is a great canvas to experiment with all types of Mediterranean ingredients and spices, as we do here with olive oil, Italian white beans, and the Middle Eastern staple spice za'atar.

Put the cannellini beans in a large bowl. Add 1 tablespoon of the reserved bean liquid and the avocado and smash with a fork or potato masher until it reaches the consistency you prefer. Gently stir in the tomatoes, vinegar, and za'atar.

Spread the smashed mixture onto the four pieces of toast. Drizzle each piece with oil and sprinkle with salt.

Healthy Kitchen Hack: Skip the toast and turn this spread into a "Mediterranean guacamole" as Deanna likes to do with the leftovers! Serve dip-style with pita chips. Or serve nacho-style and spread the leftovers over a baking sheet of pita chips, sprinkle with shredded cheese, then heat under the broiler for up to a minute until the cheese is melted (watch carefully to avoid burning).

1 (15-ounce) can cannellini beans, drained (liquid reserved) and rinsed

1 avocado, peeled, pitted, and chopped

1 large tomato, chopped

1 teaspoon red wine vinegar, white wine vinegar, or rice vinegar

1 teaspoon za'atar (see Hack on page 115)

4 slices whole-grain bread, toasted

1 teaspoon extra-virgin olive oil

¼ teaspoon kosher or sea salt

PER SERVING: Calories: 253; Total Fat: 10g; Saturated Fat: 1g; Cholesterol: 0mg; Sodium: 488mg; Total Carbohydrates: 33g; Fiber: 10g; Protein: 11g

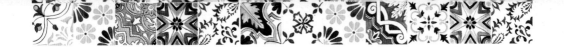

SHAKSHUKA SCRAMBLED EGGS
with Chiles

SERVES 4 Prep time: 10 minutes ✳ Cook time: 15 minutes

1 tablespoon plus
1 teaspoon extra-virgin
olive oil, divided

1 sweet bell pepper
(any color), seeded and
sliced into strips

2 garlic cloves, sliced

1 jalapeño pepper,
seeded and sliced

1 (10-ounce) can diced
tomatoes with green
chiles, drained

6 large eggs

1 teaspoon ground cumin

¼ teaspoon black pepper

½ cup chopped fresh
cilantro or parsley leaves
and stems, plus more
for garnish (optional)

3 ounces feta cheese,
crumbled (about ½ cup)

2 whole-wheat pita breads,
halved and toasted

The name "shakshuka" is likely derived from an Arab word meaning "a haphazard mixture"—and we've definitely mixed things up here! A skillet dish traditionally made of whole eggs cooked in a tomato-pepper sauce, shakshuka is popular across Libya and Tunisia and throughout the Middle East. In this sorta-spicy shakshuka-inspired dish, we use canned diced tomatoes with chiles and the eggs are scrambled instead of poached, requiring less time. Those choline-rich eggs and capsaicin-containing chiles are the perfect "wake up" for your brain health.

Heat 1 tablespoon oil in a large skillet over medium heat. Add the bell pepper, garlic, and jalapeño and cook, stirring occasionally, until they begin to soften, about 5 minutes. Add the drained tomatoes and cook, stirring occasionally until warm, about 1 minute.

While the vegetables cook, in a small bowl, whisk together the eggs, 2 tablespoons water, the cumin, and black pepper. Stir in the herbs.

Turn the heat down to medium-low. Push the vegetables to the outer edges of the skillet. Add the remaining 1 teaspoon oil and swirl it around. Pour the egg mixture into the skillet. Push in the vegetables and cook until the eggs are soft-scrambled, 4 to 6 minutes, stirring occasionally. Remove from the heat and sprinkle with the feta and, if desired, additional herbs.

Serve with the pita bread halves.

Healthy Kitchen Hack: Did you realize that the canned tomato aisle is your passport to global flavors? Along with cans of Italian-style tomatoes seasoned with garlic, oregano, and basil, there are "chili-ready" tomatoes, which are perfect for Turkish dishes because they're spiced with cumin, paprika, and chili powder. "Stewed tomatoes" often contain onions, celery, and green peppers, which work for almost any Mediterranean dish—including this shakshuka (no chopping required!). We've even found cans of French-style tomatoes with zucchini and garlic. In recipes like this one, where the tomatoes should be drained first, reserve those flavorful juices for another use, such as adding to soup broth, mixing into chili, or combining with pasta water for an instant sauce.

66

I eat eggs every morning for breakfast, but these were good enough to eat twice a day— for breakfast and dinner!

ISAAC FROM PENDLETON, OR

PER SERVING (with ½ pita): Calories: 299; Total Fat: 16g; Saturated Fat: 5g; Cholesterol: 290mg; Sodium: 711mg; Total Carbohydrates: 25g; Fiber: 3g; Protein: 16g

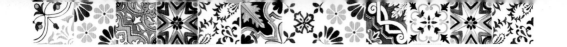

Chocolate-Tahini
POWER SHAKES

SERVES 2   Prep time: 5 minutes

1 cup 2% milk

3 Medjool dates, pitted

¾ cup plain
2% Greek yogurt or
Homemade Yogurt
(page 60)

1 tablespoon unsweetened
cocoa powder

2 teaspoons tahini

If you are a chocolate–peanut butter fan, we've got your new favorite breakfast drink! This filling shake boasts a craveable flavor combo along with brain benefits to get you through your morning routine. Tahini is a source of sesamol—a natural compound found in sesame seeds that protects against cognitive decline—while cocoa powder provides flavanols that are vital for brain function and may even improve memory.

Puree the milk and dates in a blender at high speed until the dates are pulverized (see the Hack). Add the yogurt, cocoa powder, and tahini and blend until smooth. Divide between two glasses and serve immediately.

Tip: For a fun kick (and another hit of antioxidants and aroma boosters), mix in some ground cinnamon, ginger, or nutmeg.

Healthy Kitchen Hack: During her trip to Israel, Deanna was mesmerized by the acres of date palm trees growing in the Jordan valley. Cultivated in the Middle East for thousands of years, dates are a beloved ingredient, adding natural sweetness to dishes from tagines to many regional foods and beverages. If your dates are extra-firm or a bit hard/stale, soak them in warm water for about 15 minutes to soften. Instead of storing in the pantry with other dried fruits, dates should be kept in an airtight container in the refrigerator (for up to 6 months) to maintain their moisture.

"

This shake is the perfect combination of sweet and nutty. It's very satisfying! I'd drink this for breakfast or as a filling and healthy snack.

AVA FROM
PALM BEACH, FL

PER SERVING: Calories: 260; Total Fat: 8g; Saturated Fat: 3g; Cholesterol: 18mg; Sodium: 88mg; Total Carbohydrates: 38g; Fiber: 4g; Protein: 15g

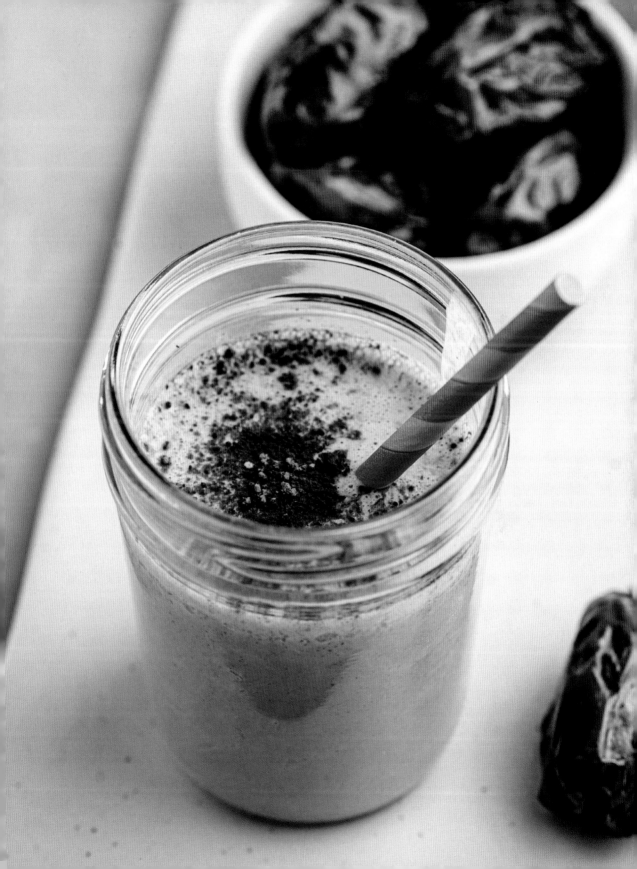

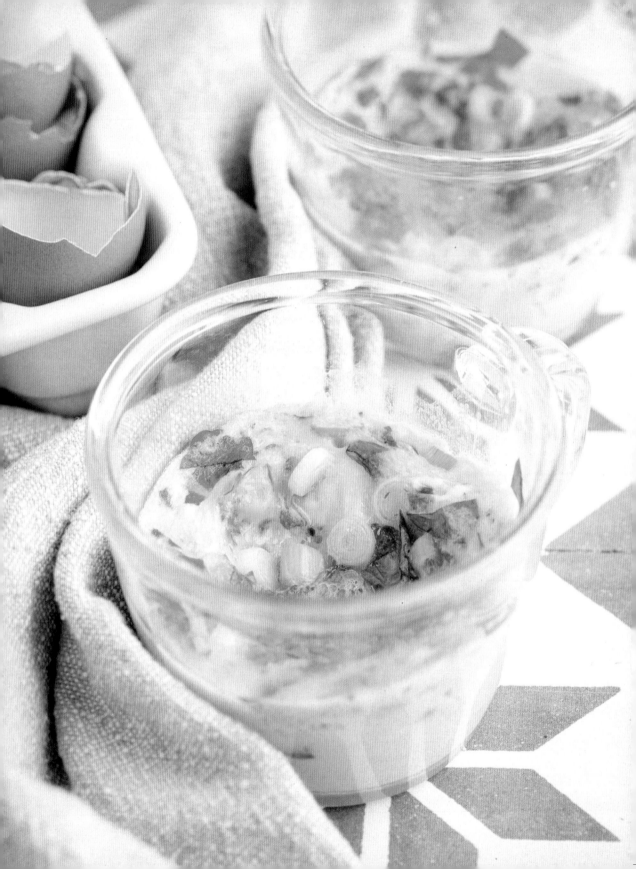

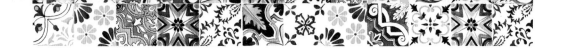

CHEESY SPINACH AND EGG MUG SCRAMBLES *with a Kick*

SERVES 2 Prep time: 5 minutes ✳ Cook time: 5 minutes

In just 10 minutes, you can fuel up with an easy egg breakfast that's rich in high-quality protein. This spinach and egg combo means a double dose of lutein and zeaxanthin—nutrients that act as internal "sunglasses" to help prevent blue light damage to the eyes from computer and phone screens, which in turn may protect your brain.

½ cup chopped
fresh spinach

1 scallion (green onion),
green and white parts,
thinly sliced

3 large eggs

1 tablespoon grated
Parmesan cheese

⅛ teaspoon crushed red
pepper, plus more for
topping (optional)

⅛ teaspoon kosher
or sea salt

Coat the inside of two coffee mugs with cooking spray. Divide the spinach and scallions between the mugs.

In a small bowl, whisk together the eggs, cheese, red pepper, salt, and 2 tablespoons water. Divide the mixture between the mugs and mix to combine.

Place both mugs in the microwave and cook, uncovered, on high for 1 minute. Stir, cover, and microwave for an additional 45 to 50 seconds, until the eggs are almost set. (The eggs will continue to cook after removing them from the microwave.) Let sit for 5 minutes to cool and finish setting.

Sprinkle with more red pepper, if desired.

Tip: Switch up this recipe by swapping in any leftover greens or herbs you may have on hand, like arugula, kale, cilantro, or parsley, and experiment with different Mediterranean spices like ground cumin, turmeric, or za'atar.

Healthy Kitchen Hack: Double or triple this recipe and freeze the extras for future breakfasts. Remove the egg scrambles from the mugs and cool. Wrap in parchment paper and then freeze in an airtight container. To reheat, microwave 2 scrambles on 50 percent power for about 1 minute. For a grab-and-go breakfast sandwich, pop the warm egg scramble between 2 pieces of whole-grain toast, a whole-grain English muffin, or a corn tortilla.

PER SERVING:
Calories: 161, Total Fat:
13g; Saturated Fat: 4g;
Cholesterol: 281mg;
Sodium: 240mg;
Total Carbohydrates: 1g;
Fiber: 0g; Protein: 11g

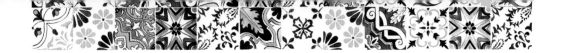

Mediterranean
SUN GOLD GRANOLA

SERVES 10 (makes about 6 cups) Prep time: 10 minutes ✳ Cook time: 30 minutes

½ cup extra-virgin olive oil

½ cup honey

1 tablespoon vanilla extract

1½ teaspoons
ground ginger

¼ teaspoon kosher
or sea salt

2 cups old-fashioned
rolled oats

1 cup sunflower seeds,
pumpkin seeds, pistachios,
chopped walnuts, or a
combination

½ cup chopped
dried apricots

½ cup golden raisins

Say good morning to this fruit-studded granola that's so tasty you'll want to eat it by the handful. If you've ever found granola a bit too crunchy for your liking, you'll love the textures in this recipe: mostly soft and chewy large chunks, with a few crispy edges. Serena's daughter said, "Mom, this granola tastes like mini oatmeal raisin cookies!" And the sweet ginger scent will do more than wake up your taste buds. In one research study, daily doses of ginger extract seemed to help women perform better in memory tests; you certainly won't forget the taste of this granola! Eat it as is, or with milk or yogurt.

Preheat the oven to 325°F. Line a large rimmed baking sheet with a sheet of parchment paper, then coat with cooking spray.

In a large bowl, whisk together the oil, honey, vanilla, ginger, and salt. Add the oats, seeds, and apricots and stir until combined. Pour onto the lined baking sheet and spread out evenly. Using a spatula or your hands, press the granola down in an even layer (depending on the size of your pan, it may not fill the entire tray; if you spread it out too much, the granola will end up very crunchy, and chewier granola is the goal!). Bake for 15 minutes, rotate the pan, and bake for another 15 to 20 minutes, until just beginning to look golden (it will still be very moist). Remove from the oven and scatter the raisins over the hot granola, then use a silicone spatula (to prevent burning your fingers) to gently press the raisins into the granola. (If you add the raisins with the apricots before baking, they can burn.)

❝

**I loved that
something so tasty
and easy required no
special ingredients
or equipment!**

MARGARET FROM
CANTON, SD

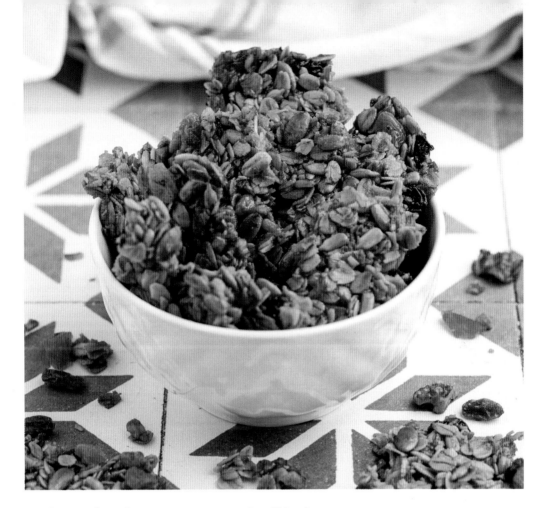

Let the granola cool to room temperature (it will harden but still be sticky) and then break the chewy granola into chunks. Serve right away, or store in an airtight container at room temperature for up to 3 days or in the freezer for up to 6 months.

Healthy Kitchen Hack: We love both Mediterranean (Turkish) apricots and California apricots, and either will work in this recipe. Mediterranean apricots are first dried whole and then pitted, while California apricots are pitted, halved, and then dried. If you use the moister Mediterranean apricots here, their plumpness may dampen the granola if stored at room temperature, so freeze it instead.

PER SERVING (about ⅔ cup): Calories: 348; Total Fat: 19g; Saturated Fat: 3g; Cholesterol: 0mg; Sodium: 61mg; Total Carbohydrates: 40g; Fiber: 4g; Protein: 5g

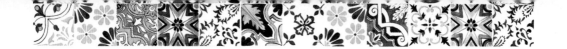

On-the-Go Breakfast
FLATBREAD WRAPS

SERVES 6   Prep time: 20 minutes ✳ Cook time: 20 minutes

1 cup instant brown rice

1 tablespoon + 1 teaspoon extra-virgin olive oil, divided

1 sweet bell pepper (any color), seeded and chopped

2 garlic cloves, minced

1 teaspoon ground cumin

¼–½ teaspoon smoked paprika

¼ teaspoon black pepper

1 (15-ounce) can chickpeas, drained (liquid reserved) and rinsed

4 ounces feta cheese, crumbled (about ⅔ cup)

¾ cup hummus (see Hack on page 157)

6 (12 × 19-inch) pieces lavash or other flatbread

Some recent studies show the brain exhibits less anxiety when it's fueled with fiber-rich foods, so invite some calm into your hectic morning routine with these Mediterranean-inspired breakfast wraps stuffed with beans, rice, and veggies. Mix them up with different spices, whole grains, and beans for a customized to-go order. See our make-ahead option below for an almost zero-stress breakfast.

Preheat the oven to 400°F. Coat a large rimmed baking sheet with cooking spray.

Cook the rice according to the package directions. Set aside.

About 5 minutes before the rice is done, heat 1 tablespoon oil in a large skillet over medium heat. Add the bell pepper and garlic and cook, stirring occasionally, until the vegetables begin to soften, about 3 minutes. Add the cumin, smoked paprika, and black pepper and cook, stirring, until the spices become fragrant, another 2 minutes. Add the chickpeas, ¼ cup of the reserved chickpea liquid, and the cooked rice and cook until heated through, stirring occasionally, 2 to 3 minutes more. Remove from the heat and stir in the cheese.

To make the wraps, spread 2 tablespoons hummus on the shorter side of the lavash, about 2 inches from the edge, then top with ⅔ cup of the rice mixture. Fold in both long sides, then fold up the bottom and roll up the lavash, sealing the edge by dipping your finger in the reserved chickpea liquid and then running it along the edge. Transfer to the prepared baking sheet, seam side down. Repeat with the remaining pieces of lavash and the filling, leaving as much room as possible between the wraps on the baking sheet. (You will have extra filling, which is delicious served on its own, stirred into soup, or used for our Green Couscous Lettuce Scoops, page 72.) Brush the tops of the wraps with the remaining 1 teaspoon oil.

Bake until the lavash is crispy, 8 to 10 minutes. Or you can skip the baking step and eat the wraps right away, but we recommend it if you like your wraps toasted and crispy like we do.

Tip: If you're serving these wraps for brunch or even dinner, consider making a batch of our tasty 10-minute Red Pepper Sauce (page 155) for dipping.

Healthy Kitchen Hack: To freeze these flatbreads, wrap each wrap individually in aluminum foil and then place in an airtight container. To reheat, place the wraps (in the aluminum foil) in a 350°F oven for 30 to 40 minutes. Or remove the wraps from the foil and microwave on defrost for about 1 minute, and then on high for about 30 seconds, until hot.

PER SERVING: Calories: 426; Total Fat: 16g; Saturated Fat: 4g; Cholesterol: 17mg; Sodium: 959mg; Total Carbohydrates: 54g; Fiber: 12g; Protein: 24g

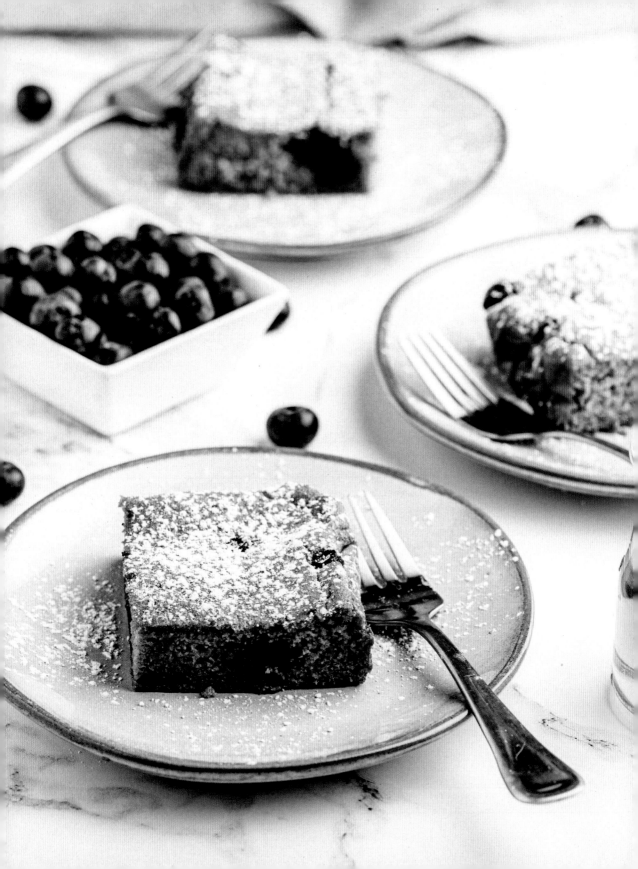

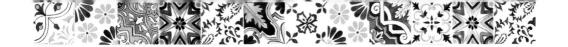

Olive Oil Berry
BREAKFAST CAKE

SERVES 9 Prep time: 25 minutes ✳ Cook time: 1 hour 10 minutes

Rise and shine with a dose of extra-virgin olive oil and your mood might be better. Emerging clinical research has shown that about 1½ tablespoons of olive oil per day can have antidepressant effects. Not to mention, waking up to the aroma of this blueberry cake baking may also boost your mood! Besides olive oil, this breakfast boasts many brain-benefiting Mediterranean ingredients, including blueberries, quinoa, cinnamon, and eggs, to start your morning off in the right direction.

Preheat the oven to 350°F. Coat a 9 × 13-inch baking pan with cooking spray.

Rinse the quinoa in a fine-mesh strainer, swirling with your fingers to wash away the bitter-tasting seed coating. Put the quinoa in a medium saucepan and cover with 1⅓ cups water. Cover the pan and bring to a boil over high heat. Lower the heat to medium and cook for 15 minutes. Turn off the heat and let the quinoa steam, still covered, for 5 more minutes, until tender. Spread the quinoa on a plate to cool for 15 to 20 minutes.

Put half of the quinoa in a food processor or blender and add the milk. Blend until smooth, then scrape down the sides. Add the remaining quinoa and 2 eggs and process until very smooth, about 1 minute. Add the remaining 2 eggs, honey, oil, baking powder, cinnamon, vanilla, baking soda, and salt. Process until smooth, about 1 minute.

⅔ cup quinoa

⅓ cup 2% milk

4 large eggs

½ cup honey

⅓ cup extra-virgin olive oil

2 teaspoons baking powder

1¼ teaspoons ground cinnamon

1 teaspoon vanilla extract

½ teaspoon baking soda

¼ teaspoon kosher or sea salt

1 cup fresh or frozen blueberries

2 tablespoons powdered sugar

continued on page 44

continued from page 43

Pour the batter into the prepared baking dish and sprinkle evenly with the blueberries. Bake for 40 to 45 minutes, until an inserted toothpick comes out nearly clean. (Avoid overbaking.) Serve warm or at room temperature, dusted with powdered sugar.

Store in an airtight container at room temperature for 1 day or in the refrigerator for up to 3 days.

Healthy Kitchen Hack: For busy mornings, prep the batter for this cake the night before. Blend up all the ingredients except the baking powder, baking soda, and blueberries. Store in a covered bowl overnight in the fridge. In the morning, whisk in the remaining ingredients, pour into the baking dish, and pop it into the oven. Adding the leavening agents (baking powder and baking soda) right before baking prevents the batter from prematurely starting to bubble and rise.

PER SERVING: Calories: 231; Total Fat: 11g; Saturated Fat: 2g; Cholesterol: 83mg; Sodium: 163mg; Total Carbohydrates: 30g; Fiber: 2g; Protein: 5g

Nutmeg
OATMEAL CUSTARD

SERVES 4   Prep time: 10 minutes ✳ Cook time: 15 minutes

The warm spice nutmeg is commonly used in both sweet and savory dishes throughout the Mediterranean. Nutmeg is a seed, so it's packed with antioxidants. Even if the amounts used are small, those small amounts add up— not to mention, your brain will focus much, much better after any nourishing breakfast. This one checks all the boxes: it's quick, protein-packed, enriched with whole-grains, and "nutmeg amazing"!

4 cups 2% milk

2 cups rolled oats (old-fashioned or quick)

Grated zest of 1 lemon

½ teaspoon nutmeg, preferably freshly grated

3 large eggs

2 tablespoons honey

½ teaspoon vanilla extract

In a saucepan, combine the milk, oats, lemon zest, and nutmeg. Heat over medium-high heat until just boiling, stirring occasionally to prevent sticking on the bottom. Reduce the heat to medium. Cook, stirring frequently and scraping the bottom, until creamy, 3 to 4 minutes. Add the eggs, stirring constantly with a fork until the mixture is no longer shiny and the eggs are cooked, about 1 minute. Stir in the honey and vanilla and serve warm in individual bowls.

Healthy Kitchen Hack: To shave a few minutes off this breakfast in the morning, assemble the milk, water, oats, and nutmeg in the saucepan the night before. Refrigerate overnight. The oats will soften and reduce the cooking time—plus save the measuring time. And in the morning, every minute counts.

PER SERVING: Calories: 393; Total Fat: 9g; Saturated Fat: 5g; Cholesterol: 159mg; Sodium: 169mg; Total Carbohydrates: 53g; Fiber: 5g; Protein: 19g

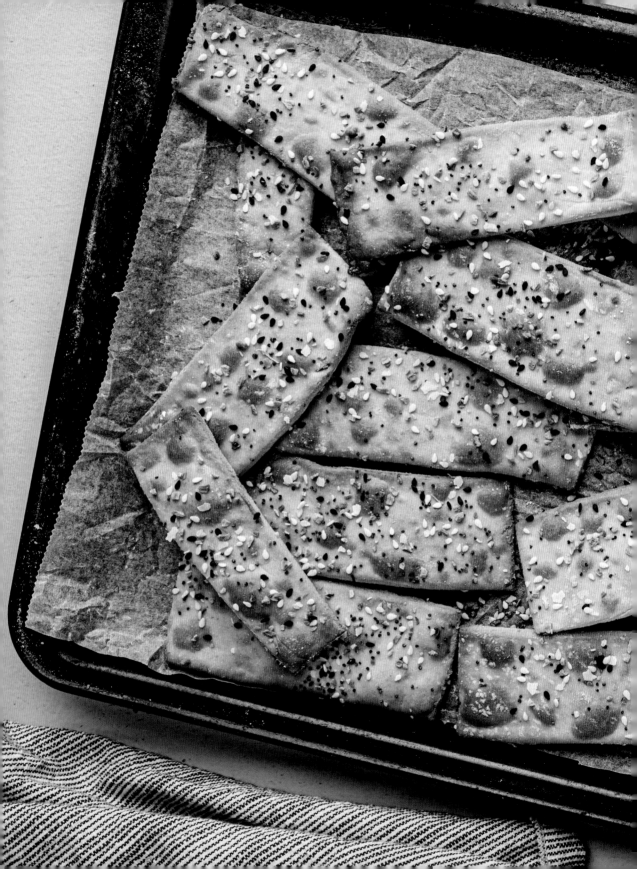

SMALL PLATES & SNACKS

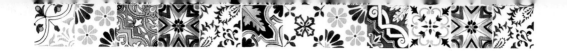

Honey-Turmeric
SALTED PEANUTS

SERVES 6 Prep time: 5 minutes ❋ Cook time: 5 minutes

1½ cups unsalted
dry-roasted peanuts

¼ teaspoon kosher
or sea salt

¼ teaspoon black pepper

1 tablespoon honey

1 teaspoon ground
turmeric

Turmeric, the gorgeous yellow-orange spice that's ubiquitous in Middle Eastern and North African cuisines, has potent protective properties. Some research suggests it can slow down the natural death of brain cells and even stop unnatural cell death from toxins, trauma, and infections. But curcuminoids—the antioxidants in turmeric—can slightly degrade with cooking, reducing some (but not all!) of their powerful capabilities. Here, the turmeric only warms for a minute to keep its potency, turning plain peanuts into a snack with serious cred in terms of salty-sweet-peppery yumminess, and in brain-boosting benefits.

Lay a piece of parchment paper on a rimmed baking sheet or heat-proof surface.

In a large skillet on a cold stove, combine the peanuts, salt, and pepper. Turn the heat to medium. Stir frequently until the nuts are warm, about 2 minutes.

Add the honey and turmeric and cook, stirring frequently, until the nuts are completely coated, 1 to 2 minutes (be careful not to burn the nuts, as they brown quickly). Remove from the heat and carefully spread the nuts on the parchment paper. Cool completely, at least 15 minutes (the nuts will still be somewhat sticky). Store the nuts in an airtight container at room temperature for up to a week, or in the freezer for longer storage.

PER SERVING: Calories: 227; Total Fat: 18g; Saturated Fat: 3g; Cholesterol: 0mg; Sodium: 83mg; Total Carbohydrates: 11g; Fiber: 3g; Protein: 9g

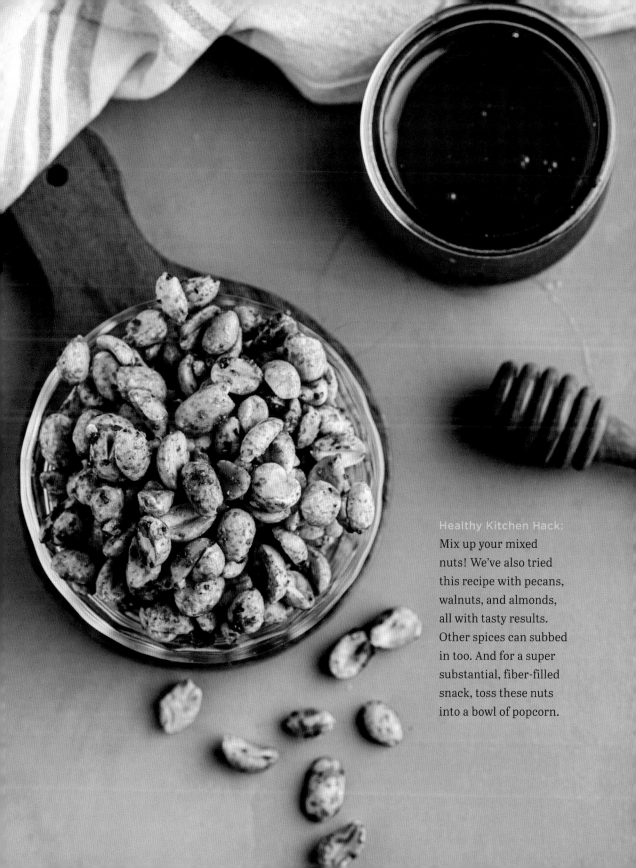

Healthy Kitchen Hack:
Mix up your mixed
nuts! We've also tried
this recipe with pecans,
walnuts, and almonds,
all with tasty results.
Other spices can subbed
in too. And for a super
substantial, fiber-filled
snack, toss these nuts
into a bowl of popcorn.

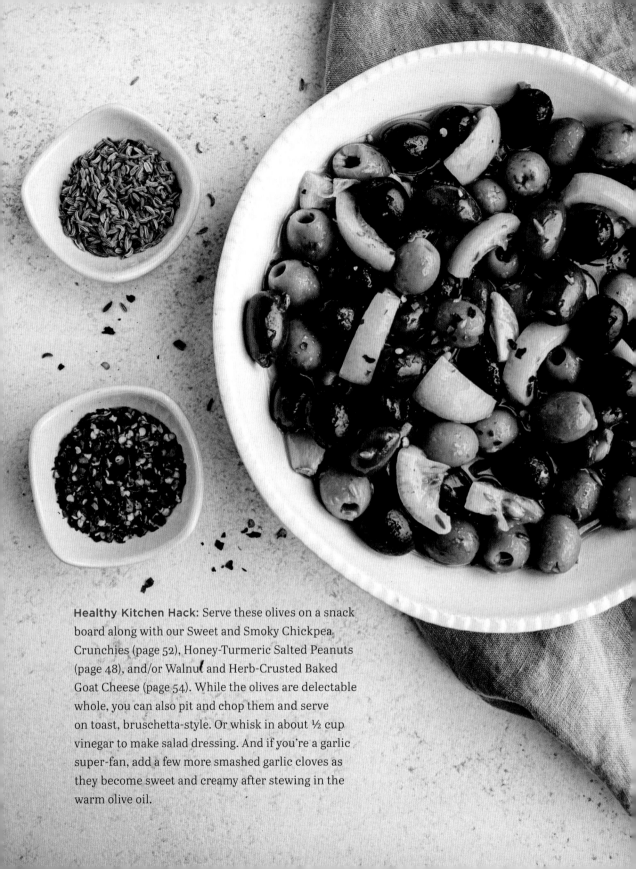

Healthy Kitchen Hack: Serve these olives on a snack board along with our Sweet and Smoky Chickpea Crunchies (page 52), Honey-Turmeric Salted Peanuts (page 48), and/or Walnut and Herb-Crusted Baked Goat Cheese (page 54). While the olives are delectable whole, you can also pit and chop them and serve on toast, bruschetta-style. Or whisk in about ½ cup vinegar to make salad dressing. And if you're a garlic super-fan, add a few more smashed garlic cloves as they become sweet and creamy after stewing in the warm olive oil.

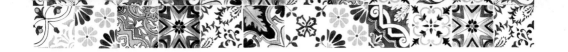

Marvelous
MEDITERRANEAN OLIVES

SERVES 8   Prep time: 10 minutes   ✳   Cook time: 10 minutes

We're doubling down on our olive love with these irresistible buttery olives marinated in olive oil infused with lemon, black and red pepper, and garlic. Which means twice the brain benefits from both the depression-fighting components of olive oil and the fiber- and antioxidant-rich olives themselves. While these olives feel fancy, they are super simple to whip up. Enjoy them with some crusty bread to sop up the extra flavorful oil (and for more serving ideas, see the Hack).

⅔ cup extra-virgin olive oil

5 garlic cloves,
lightly smashed

½ lemon, thinly sliced

1 teaspoon fennel seeds

¼ teaspoon crushed
red pepper

¼ teaspoon black pepper

2½ cups mixed black
and green olives
(such as Kalamata,
Castelvetrano, Niçoise,
canned California green,
and/or canned black)

Heat the oil in a small saucepan over medium heat. Add the garlic and lemon and cook, stirring occasionally, until the mixture sizzles and the garlic begins to turn golden, 7 to 10 minutes. Remove from the heat and stir in the fennel, red pepper, and black pepper. Let cool for about 10 minutes.

Spoon the olives into a wide, flat serving dish or, if making ahead, into a 2-quart jar. Pour the warm olive oil mixture over the olives and stir gently to combine (or close the jar lid and shake gently).

Serve immediately or after marinating for up to 4 hours at room temperature. If making ahead, the olives can be refrigerated for up to 2 weeks and brought to room temperature before serving.

PER SERVING: Calories: 217; Total Fat: 23g; Saturated Fat: 3g; Cholesterol: 0mg; Sodium: 310mg; Total Carbohydrates: 5g; Fiber: 2g; Protein: 1g

Sweet and Smoky
CHICKPEA CRUNCHIES

SERVES 4   Prep time: 5 minutes   ✳   Cook time: 25 minutes

1 (15-ounce) can chickpeas, drained and rinsed

1 tablespoon extra-virgin olive oil

1 teaspoon sugar

½ teaspoon unsweetened cocoa powder

½ teaspoon smoked paprika

⅛ teaspoon kosher or sea salt

From hummus to falafel to socca, dishes from countries throughout the Mediterranean feature chickpeas, so we always have this ubiquitous staple ingredient in our pantries. And if you've never sampled them crunchy, get ready for your new favorite smarter snack. Loaded with fiber, iron, B vitamins, and magnesium, legumes like chickpeas deliver a slew of brain benefits when consumed daily. And the combo of cocoa, smoked paprika, salt, and sugar hits every taste bud on your tongue!

Preheat the oven to 450°F. Pat the chickpeas dry on a kitchen towel, then place them on a large rimmed baking sheet. Drizzle the oil over them, then sprinkle with the sugar, cocoa powder, smoked paprika, and salt. Using your hands, toss all the ingredients together until the chickpeas are thoroughly coated. Spread them out on the sheet. Bake for 10 minutes, then, using an oven mitt, shake the pan a few times to move them around. Continue to bake for another 12 to 14 minutes, until the chickpeas are golden and crispy.

Cool slightly before serving.

Tip: Enjoy these chickpeas the day you make them as they get less crispy over time. If you have leftovers, store them at room temperature in a loosely covered container or bowl for up to 3 days. To recrisp, heat the chickpeas under the broiler for 30 to 60 seconds—be careful not to let them burn!

Healthy Kitchen Hack: Besides swapping in different dried herbs and spices to change up the flavor profile, make your own brain-booster snack mix by combining these crunchy chickpeas with a few cups of popcorn (a whole grain), a handful of your favorite nuts, and dried berries or raisins.

PER SERVING: Calories: 134; Total Fat: 6g; Saturated Fat: 1g; Cholesterol: 0mg; Sodium: 163mg; Total Carbohydrates: 16g; Fiber: 5g; Protein: 6g

North African
SWEET HOT PEPPER PICKLES

SERVES 10   Prep time: 15 minutes, plus 2 hours refrigeration   ✳ Cook time: 5 minutes

Pickles can make bland food taste better, cut the richness of heavy foods, and add the "sparkle" of acid to just about any savory dish. Enjoying these quick fresh veggie pickles is an easy way to increase your fiber intake—and higher fiber diets are tied to less anxiety. Inspired by the flavors of Morocco, Algeria, and Tunisia, these pickles can be made from just about any vegetable, including cauliflower, carrots, cucumbers, bell peppers, green beans, cherry tomatoes, red onion rings, beets, and okra. Serve with a bowl of couscous as is routine in these North African countries or pair them with almost any savory dish in this book—they're that versatile.

5 cups cut vegetables of choice (see headnote)

2 (4-inch) Anaheim peppers, seeded and sliced into strips (see Tip)

2 garlic cloves, lightly smashed

3 cups white wine vinegar or apple cider vinegar

¼ cup sugar

3 tablespoons kosher or sea salt

1 tablespoon coriander seeds or 3 tablespoons chopped fresh cilantro stems

1 teaspoon cumin seeds or ground cumin

¼ teaspoon Urfa or Aleppo chile flakes or crushed red pepper

¼ teaspoon black pepper, preferably freshly ground

Divide the vegetable pieces and peppers into 2 quart-size mason jars or put them all in a large, heatproof glass bowl. Add one garlic clove to each jar, or put both in the bowl.

In a medium saucepan, combine 3 cups water, the vinegar, sugar, salt, coriander, cumin, chile flakes, and black pepper and stir together. Bring to a boil over medium-high heat, stirring occasionally. Carefully pour the hot brine over the vegetables. Refrigerate the pickles for at least 2 hours. Enjoy them right out of the jars, or cover and keep refrigerated for up to 2 weeks.

Tip: Instead of Anaheim peppers, try jalapeños for more heat, or 1 large bell pepper for less heat.

Healthy Kitchen Hack: Reuse that flavorful pickle liquid! After your pickles are gone, add a new batch of veggies to the pickle liquid and refrigerate overnight. After those pickles are gone, use the leftover liquid to make homemade salad dressing by whisking with an equal amount of olive oil, Greek yogurt, or mayonnaise.

PER SERVING:
Calories: 30; Total Fat: 0g;
Saturated Fat: 0g;
Cholesterol: 0mg;
Sodium: 160mg;
Total Carbohydrates:
7g; Fiber: 1g; Protein: 1g
(Note: Nutritional values
will vary depending on
vegetables used.)

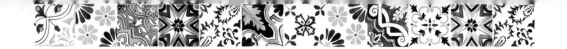

Walnut and Herb-Crusted
BAKED GOAT CHEESE

SERVES 9 Prep time: 10 minutes ✳ Cook time: 10 minutes

½ cup chopped walnuts

¼ cup finely chopped fresh mint leaves and stems

Grated zest of 1 lemon

2 teaspoons chopped fresh chives

1 teaspoon za'atar (see Hack on page 115)

¼ teaspoon black pepper

3 (4-ounce) goat cheese logs

1½ teaspoons honey

36 multigrain crackers

1 cucumber, peeled and sliced

Instead of serving your goat cheese cold straight from the fridge, with a little bit of heat and some brain-boosting Mediterranean staples, you'll impress your guests (or yourself) with this anytime appetizer/snack. It's got brain-protective omega-3s from the walnuts, memory-improving choline plus folate from the chives, and a dash of antioxidants from the black pepper and za'atar. And breathe in the fresh mint, as studies suggest its aroma can help improve mood and mental clarity.

Preheat the oven to 375°F. Spread a sheet of parchment paper on a large rimmed baking sheet.

In a medium bowl, combine the walnuts, mint, lemon zest, chives, za'atar, and pepper and mix well. Roll and gently press one cheese log in the walnut mix until the entire log (ends, too) is covered. Place on the prepared sheet and repeat with the remaining two cheese logs. Bake for 8 to 10 minutes, until the logs are warmed through and soft when you gently press in the center.

Transfer the logs to a platter, drizzle with the honey, and serve with crackers and sliced cucumber.

Healthy Kitchen Hack: Turn a cheese log into a creamy, dreamy pasta sauce. Bake one of the encrusted logs for an additional 3 to 5 minutes, until the goat cheese just starts to ooze. Scrape it into a small saucepan over low heat and whisk in 4 to 5 tablespoons warm milk or the starchy water from cooking pasta. Toss with about 4 cups cooked pasta (approximately 8 ounces uncooked) and top with additional herbs.

PER SERVING (⅓ log with 5 cucumber slices and 4 crackers): Calories: 240; Total Fat: 15g; Saturated Fat: 6g; Cholesterol: 17mg; Sodium: 445mg; Total Carbohydrates: 18g; Fiber: 2g; Protein: 10g

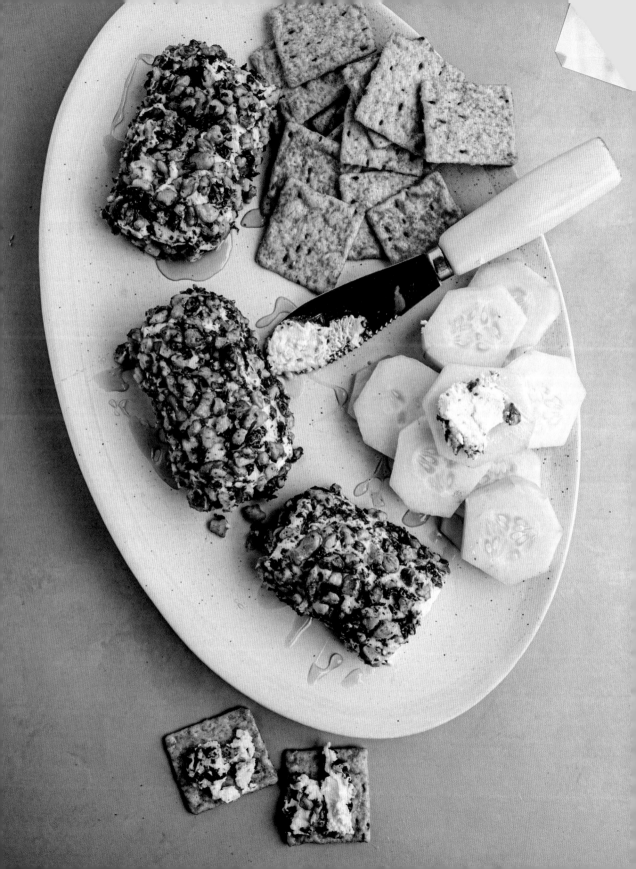

Healthy Kitchen Hack: Turn this dip into dinner! Spread the prepared dip on a platter and top with cooked shrimp, scallops, ground beef, or tofu. Top with the parsley and pomegranate seeds, if desired, and serve with additional pita bread.

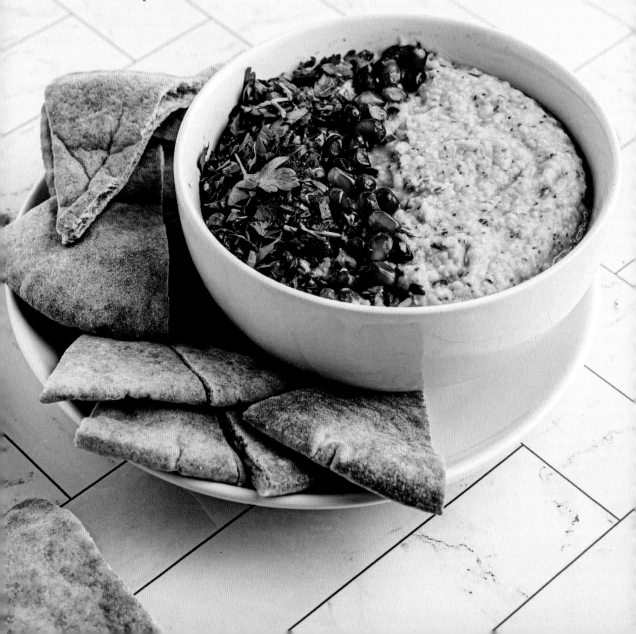

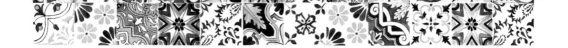

BABY LIMA BEAN DIP
with Parsley and Pomegranate

SERVES 8 (makes about 2¾ cups) Prep time: 10 minutes ❋ Cook time: 5 minutes

Deanna was giddy when her friend Nicole lent her a cookbook by her Syrian grandmother, which was published by her New Jersey–based church back in the '70s. Cookin' Good with Sitto *features "traditional Mid-Eastern recipes" handed down from generations, after coming to America. This appetizer is a riff on Sitto's "Fool Em-dam-mas" (ful medames, an Egyptian and Middle Eastern fava bean dip). We swapped in frozen baby lima beans for the canned favas, which can be hard to find. But whether limas, favas, or butter beans, these legumes provide the brain with vital amino acids, vitamins, and minerals including a hefty dose of folate, which is crucial to warding off neurovegetative diseases. Bonus: the original dip and this version also include a pretty pop of red from pomegranate seeds.*

1 (1-pound) bag frozen baby lima beans

1 lemon

⅓ cup fresh parsley leaves and stems, plus more for garnish

2 tablespoons extra-virgin olive oil

2 garlic cloves, peeled

½ teaspoon smoked paprika

¼ teaspoon kosher or sea salt

¼ teaspoon black pepper

¼ cup pomegranate seeds

4 whole-wheat pita breads, cut into triangles

Cook the baby lima beans in water (typically about ½ cup) according to the package directions.

Transfer the cooked beans with the cooking water to a blender or food processor. Using a Microplane or citrus zester, grate the zest from the lemon into the blender, then cut the lemon in half and squeeze in the juice. Add the parsley, oil, garlic, smoked paprika, salt, and pepper. Pour in ½ cup fresh water and start to puree. Add more water, 1 tablespoon at a time, until the puree reaches a hummus-like consistency.

Spoon the bean dip into a medium bowl. Sprinkle with additional chopped parsley and pomegranate seeds. Serve with pita bread.

PER SERVING (about ⅓ cup dip with ½ pita bread): Calories: 197; Total Fat: 4g; Saturated Fat: 1g; Cholesterol: 0mg; Sodium: 260mg; Total Carbohydrates: 34g; Fiber: 6g; Protein: 8g

Cumin-Sesame
CHICKPEA CRACKERS

SERVES 8–10 (makes about 36 crackers) Prep time: 30 minutes ✳ Cook time: 15 minutes

3 cups chickpea flour

2 tablespoons plus
1 teaspoon everything
bagel seasoning, divided
(see Hack)

1 teaspoon honey

¾ teaspoon ground cumin

¼ teaspoon kosher
or sea salt

¼ teaspoon black pepper

3 tablespoons extra-virgin
olive oil

> 66
>
> **These crackers
> were surprisingly
> easy to make and
> the simple dough
> makes it possible
> for a multitude of
> variations.**
>
> AILEEN FROM
> WARRINGTON, PA

If you can bake cookies, you can bake these irresistible gluten-free crackers! Studded with seeds, garlic, salt, and pepper, these crunchers are made with chickpea flour (also known as garbanzo bean flour or gram flour)—a good source of magnesium, which is vital for memory and mental health. Serve them with dip like our Baby Lima Bean Dip with Parsley and Pomegranate (page 57), soup like our Spicy Turmeric Chicken Minestrone Soup (page 101), or break them up over a salad as instant croutons.

Preheat the oven to 400°F. Line two large rimmed baking sheets with parchment paper.

In a large mixing bowl or stand mixer, mix the flour, 1 teaspoon everything bagel seasoning, honey, cumin, salt, and pepper. Mix in the oil with ⅔ cup water, a few tablespoons at a time, until a slightly sticky dough forms. Transfer the dough to a lightly chickpea flour–dusted work surface and dust the top of the dough with flour, too. Knead for 1 to 2 minutes until smooth (if the dough is too sticky when kneading, add a few more teaspoons of flour to the work surface and work it in). Divide into two portions.

Take the parchment paper off a baking sheet and dust the parchment with flour. Place one of the dough portions on it. With a flour-dusted rolling pin, roll the dough into a 12-inch square about ⅛ inch thick. Dust the dough with flour if it gets too sticky to roll. Place the parchment with the rolled-out dough back on the baking sheet. Using a pizza cutter or sharp knife, cut into 1½ × 4-inch strips (to make this process easier, you can make a template with a piece of paper).

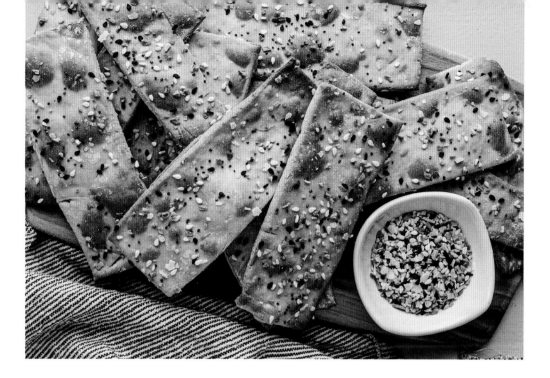

Separate and make a little bit of room between each cracker strip. Add any leftover cut dough scraps to the remaining dough portion and repeat the process with the other baking sheet.

Lightly brush the crackers with water and sprinkle with the remaining 2 tablespoons everything bagel seasoning. Bake for 12 to 15 minutes, until golden brown, rotating and swapping the sheets halfway during baking. Remove the sheets and carefully transfer each parchment paper to cooling racks (the crackers will continue to crisp as they cool). Store crackers in an airtight container in the pantry for up to 5 days.

Healthy Kitchen Hack: Deanna uses everything bagel seasoning in just about…everything! But if you don't have it on hand, swap in 1¼ teaspoons sesame seeds, 1¼ teaspoons poppy seeds, ¼ teaspoon garlic powder, and ¼ teaspoon kosher or sea salt for every 1 tablespoon. Or, as we routinely encourage our readers, experiment with different spices (antioxidant powerhouses!) from your spice drawer—like fennel seeds, Italian seasoning, or even cinnamon sugar— in the dough and on top.

PER SERVING
(4 crackers): Calories: 162;
Total Fat: 7g;
Saturated Fat: 1g;
Cholesterol: 0mg;
Sodium: 273mg;
Total Carbohydrates: 19g;
Fiber: 3g; Protein: 7g

HOMEMADE YOGURT

SERVES 7 (makes about 5 cups)   Prep time: 45 minutes ✳ Cook time: 24 hours

5¼ cups whole milk

3 tablespoons whole-milk plain yogurt (see Tip)

Prepare to have your mind blown! Not only will you be surprised how easy it is to make cool, creamy homemade yogurt (basically by extending a small amount of store-bought yogurt), but also you might not know that the thinner "regular" yogurt is much more common in the Mediterranean than the thicker, strained Greek style. You can make both styles with this recipe. We typically use Greek yogurt because its higher protein content increases the protein in plant-based recipes. But if we're spooning up this velvety homemade yogurt topped with honey and nuts, we generally eat it without straining, and still get all the good nutrients and probiotics for brain and mind well-being.

66

I can't believe I can make great yogurt at home that in the store would have cost me around $10!

BONNIE FROM
MANHATTAN, MT

Note: To make this recipe, you will need some specific equipment. Have ready 3 (1-pint) mason jars with lids, a large stockpot, clean dishcloths, a digital thermometer, rubber dishwashing gloves or canning jar pinchers, and a hard-sided plastic cooler (any size) or a 7-quart slow cooker. Sterilize the mason jars, lids, and a fork in the dishwasher or wash with hot soapy water and allow them to air-dry so they are free of bacteria.

Place a dishcloth in the stockpot to keep the jars from knocking together during heating. Fill the stockpot with about 2 inches of water and place on the stove; check to make sure that all three jars fit inside the pot and that the water comes to within 1–2 inches of the tops of the jars. (Remove the jars to fill.)

Pour the milk into the jars so it comes to within about 1 inch of the top of each jar. Carefully place the jars in the stockpot (do not cover with the lids). Turn the heat to medium-high and bring the milk to a temperature of 180°F (it takes about 20 minutes), checking the temperature with the digital thermometer often to make sure it does not go over 190°F. Using rubber gloves or canning pinchers, carefully remove the jars and set them on a clean dishcloth on the counter (leave the water in the pot). Continuously check the temperature of the milk until it cools to 110°F—it takes about 1 hour, or you can place the jars in an ice bath for about 10 minutes, but watch carefully to prevent cooling below 110°F. Then add about 1 tablespoon yogurt to each jar of milk and stir with a sterilized fork to incorporate.

Cover the jars with the lids and transfer to the hard-sided cooler. Add the reserved (about 120°F) warm water from the stockpot to a level of about 1½ inches from the top of the jars. (Alternatively, place the jars in a slow cooker, then pour in about 2 inches of the warm pot water; place the lid on the slow cooker and turn to warm, not low.) Let the yogurt sit for 20 to 24 hours, until it is set and no longer liquidy throughout. (Some liquid whey will remain on the top; this can be stirred in or drained off—see the Hack.) Store in the refrigerator for up to 3 weeks.

Tip: Use very fresh plain yogurt and a brand whose flavor you like, either regular or Greek style. Your homemade yogurt will take on the taste of the purchased plain yogurt as the cultures will multiply in your version. You can also start with a flavored yogurt as long as it contains live active cultures, but the finished yogurt will not taste like the flavored yogurt (unless you add those desired flavors to the finished yogurt).

Healthy Kitchen Hack: Greek yogurt is thicker yogurt made by straining off the liquid whey. To make this style, strain your homemade yogurt by lining a mesh strainer or colander with paper coffee filters or cheesecloth and set in a large bowl. Spoon in the yogurt (you may have to do this in batches depending on the size of your strainer). Let the liquid whey drain out of the yogurt for at least 2 hours in the refrigerator, or longer depending on the thickness desired. To use up the leftover whey, substitute it for milk in most recipes—blend it into smoothies, mix it into pancakes, waffles, quick breads, or muffin batters, or use it for cooking oatmeal or other grains.

PER SERVING (²/₃ cup unstrained yogurt): Calories: 122; Total Fat: 6g; Saturated Fat: 3g; Cholesterol: 20mg; Sodium: 86mg; Total Carbohydrates: 10g; Fiber: 0g; Protein: 6g

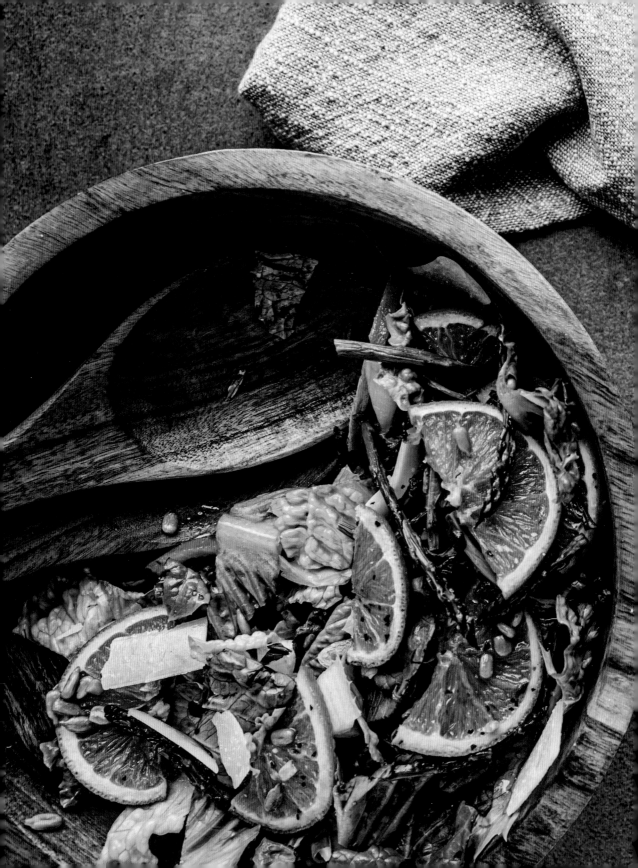

SALADS

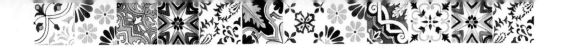

BERRY SMART SEEDED DRESSING
over Greens

SERVES 6 Prep time: 15 minutes

Berry Smart Seeded Dressing

1 cup frozen or fresh blueberries, strawberries, raspberries, and/or blackberries

1 tablespoon balsamic or white wine vinegar

1½ teaspoons honey

1 teaspoon Dijon mustard

¼ teaspoon kosher or sea salt

¼ teaspoon black pepper

3 tablespoons extra-virgin olive oil

1 tablespoon poppy or sesame seeds

Salad

8 cups spinach or other salad greens

1 cup fresh berries and/or grapes

¼ cup sunflower seeds, pepitas, pistachios, and/or chopped walnuts

2 ounces Gorgonzola, feta, or other aged cheese, crumbled (about ⅓ cup)

Happily, Serena's children will eat any salad greens drizzled with this bright, fruity dressing. Using any sweet berries you have on hand—frozen, or even fresh ones that are beginning to look shriveled—this colorful dressing brings a fresh and sweet flavor to spinach, romaine, or baby greens. Berries, leafy greens, and seeds are three of the highest rated foods for cognitive health, so adding this salad to your regular recipe routine is a no-brainer!

Put the berries, vinegar, honey, mustard, salt, and pepper in a blender and pulse until combined. With the motor running, pour in the oil and blend until smooth; add 1 to 2 tablespoons water if the dressing seems thick (this will depend on the juiciness of your berries). Add the poppy seeds and pulse once to combine.

Put the spinach, berries/grapes, sunflower seeds, and cheese in a serving bowl. Immediately before serving, pour the dressing over the salad and toss to combine, if desired.

Tip: This recipe makes about 1½ cups dressing, which is perfect for six large side salads. If you are serving fewer salads or making the dressing ahead of time, store it in the refrigerator. If using blueberries, note that they tend to gel if they sit, so you'll need to whisk in 1 tablespoon water to thin out the saved dressing.

PER SERVING: Calories: 185; Total Fat: 14g; Saturated Fat: 3g; Cholesterol: 7mg; Sodium: 261mg Total Carbohydrates: 13g; Fiber: 3g; Protein: 5g

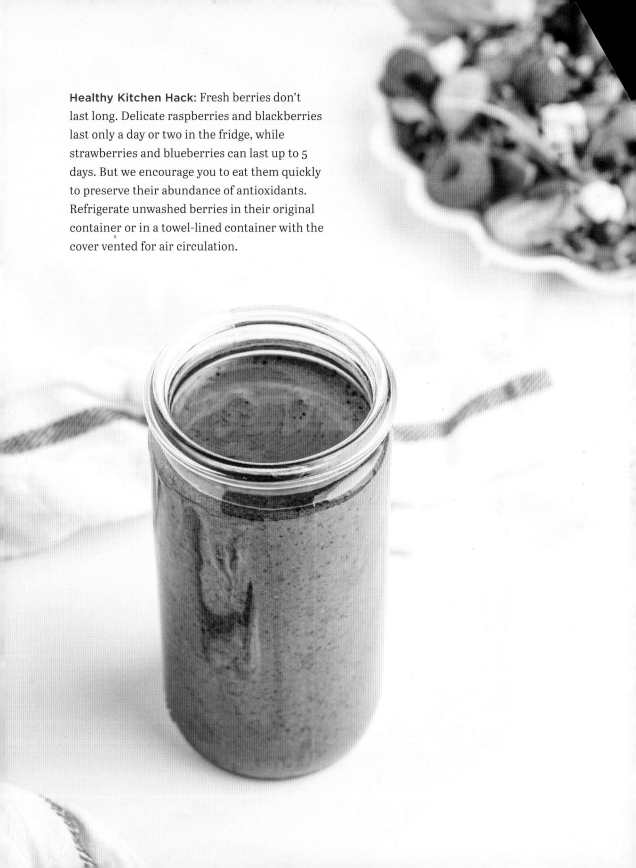

Healthy Kitchen Hack: Fresh berries don't last long. Delicate raspberries and blackberries last only a day or two in the fridge, while strawberries and blueberries can last up to 5 days. But we encourage you to eat them quickly to preserve their abundance of antioxidants. Refrigerate unwashed berries in their original container or in a towel-lined container with the cover vented for air circulation.

CREAMY CUCUMBER SALAD
with Sesame Dressing

SERVES 4   Prep time: 15 minutes

3 scallions (green onions), green and white parts, sliced, divided

3 tablespoons plain whole-milk Greek yogurt or Homemade Yogurt (page 60)

1 tablespoon tahini

1 tablespoon white wine vinegar or other vinegar

2 teaspoons extra-virgin olive oil

½ teaspoon kosher or sea salt

¼ teaspoon black pepper

2 cucumbers, cut into ¼-inch-thick slices

1 tablespoon toasted sesame seeds (see Hack)

Looking at a map of the Mediterranean Sea, you'll see the northern part turns into the Adriatic Sea, and at the very top is the short coastline of Slovenia. Milk production is the country's largest agricultural activity, and some of that milk is made into decadent fermented dairy foods like yogurt and kefir. Serena created this recipe based on a tangy sour cream, cucumber, and onion salad that her grandmother used to make and that you may find in Slovenia. A double dose of nutty, slightly sweet sesame seeds complements the creaminess of whole-milk yogurt.

In a mini food processor or blender, combine a third of the scallion slices, the yogurt, tahini, vinegar, oil, salt, and pepper and blend until pureed.

Put the cucumber in a serving bowl. Add the remaining scallions and the dressing and toss to combine. Sprinkle the salad with the toasted sesame seeds and serve.

Healthy Kitchen Hack: Toasted sesame seeds add nutty zip to any salad, yogurt parfait, or soup. Put about ¼ cup sesame seeds in a dry skillet and cook over medium-low heat, stirring occasionally, for 2 to 3 minutes, until very fragrant. Store leftovers in an airtight container at room temperature for up to a week or in the refrigerator for up to 3 months.

PER SERVING: Calories: 109; Total Fat: 8g; Saturated Fat: 1g; Cholesterol: 2mg; Sodium: 165mg; Total Carbohydrates: 8g; Fiber: 1g; Protein: 3g

September
APPLE-CELERY SALAD

SERVES 6 Prep time: 20 minutes

Serena grew up on a farm in Montana, and every September her grandmother would make a salad similar to this one with apples from their orchard. Serena now makes it for her family where they live in the countryside outside St. Louis, using apples from her own three little apple trees. We envision that the grandmothers in northern Greece, where apples grow, may also make salads like this one, which sings with contrasting flavors of sweet fruit, salty feta, grassy parsley, and acidic lemon. Every ingredient in this salad can aid in brain health, wherever you eat it.

Using a Microplane or citrus zester, grate the zest from the lemon into a large serving bowl, then cut the lemon in half and squeeze in 1 tablespoon juice (save the remaining lemon for another use). Whisk in the oil, honey, salt, and red pepper. Add the celery, parsley, and apples and toss well to coat. Add the almonds and cheese, toss gently, and serve.

Healthy Kitchen Hack: For crisper, crunchier celery in any salad, sandwich spread, or crudité platter, hydrate it first. Our recipe testers said that without hydration, the celery was "sharp" and "spicy," but after soaking, it was "sweet" and "crisp." To hydrate, fill a large bowl with ice water, add the sliced celery, and let soak for 20 minutes. Drain, place the celery on a clean towel, and pat dry.

1 lemon

2 tablespoons extra-virgin olive oil

1 teaspoon honey

½ teaspoon kosher or sea salt

⅛–¼ teaspoon crushed red pepper

6 celery ribs with leaves, sliced diagonally into ½-inch slices (see Hack)

2 cups chopped fresh parsley leaves and stems

3 apples, unpeeled, cored, and chopped

⅓ cup chopped almonds, pistachios, sunflower seeds, pepitas, and/or other nuts or seeds

2 ounces feta cheese, crumbled (about ⅓ cup)

PER SERVING: Calories: 180; Total Fat: 11g; Saturated Fat: 3g; Cholesterol: 8mg; Sodium: 254mg; Total Carbohydrates: 19g; Fiber: 5g; Protein: 4g

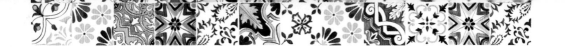

Roasted ORANGE, ASPARAGUS, AND PARMESAN SALAD

SERVES 8 Prep time: 15 minutes ✳ Cook time: 15 minutes

1 pound asparagus, trimmed

2 oranges, unpeeled, halved, and very thinly sliced

5 tablespoons extra-virgin olive oil, divided

½ teaspoon kosher or sea salt, divided

½ teaspoon black pepper, divided

¼ cup orange juice

1 tablespoon honey

1 tablespoon red wine vinegar, white wine vinegar, or rice vinegar

½ teaspoon ground ginger

2 heads romaine lettuce, chopped (about 10 cups)

¾ cup shaved Parmesan cheese (about 3 ounces)

2 tablespoons chopped fresh chives or scallions (green onions), green and white parts

2 tablespoons sunflower seeds

Deanna calls this her "transition to spring" salad as she makes it when asparagus season starts, hinting at the warmer and longer days to follow. Along with the mood boost of sunnier days in sight, this salad showcases green veggies, citrus, seeds, and even ginger—common Mediterranean ingredients that contribute nutrients to protect our cognitive and mental health. And yes, you can eat orange rinds, especially when roasted into tantalizing, caramelized slices.

Arrange the oven racks in the upper-middle and lower-middle positions. Preheat the oven to 450°F. Coat two large rimmed baking sheets with cooking spray or line with parchment paper.

Place the asparagus on one sheet and the orange slices on the other sheet so the pieces are not touching each other. Brush both the asparagus and the oranges with 2 tablespoons oil and sprinkle both with ¼ teaspoon salt and ¼ teaspoon pepper. Roast for 5 minutes, flip the orange slices, and switch the sheet pans' positions in the oven. Continue roasting until the asparagus is tender and the orange flesh is slightly browned, another 5 to 7 minutes. Remove from the oven and, once cooled, cut the asparagus into bite-size pieces.

While the asparagus and oranges roast, whisk the remaining 3 tablespoons oil, orange juice, honey, vinegar, ginger, and remaining ¼ teaspoon salt and ¼ teaspoon pepper in a small bowl. Set aside.

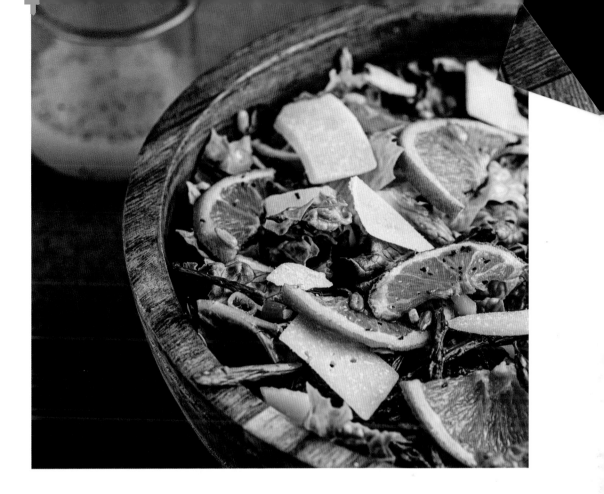

To arrange the salad, put the romaine in a large serving bowl. Add the roasted oranges, asparagus, cheese, chives, and seeds. Drizzle with the dressing, toss, and serve immediately.

Healthy Kitchen Hack: Take this salad to the next level and grill your romaine! The heat creates a lovely smoky flavor and another layer of texture. Instead of chopping, cut the romaine heads in half lengthwise, drizzle with a little of the dressing, and then place, cut side down, on the grill. Grill, uncovered, until slightly charred, 1 to 2 minutes. Chop the grilled romaine and toss with the rest of the salad ingredients, including the remaining dressing.

PER SERVING: Calories: 186; Total Fat: 13g; Saturated Fat: 3g; Cholesterol: 5mg; Sodium: 262mg; Total Carbohydrates: 16g; Fiber: 6g; Protein: 7g

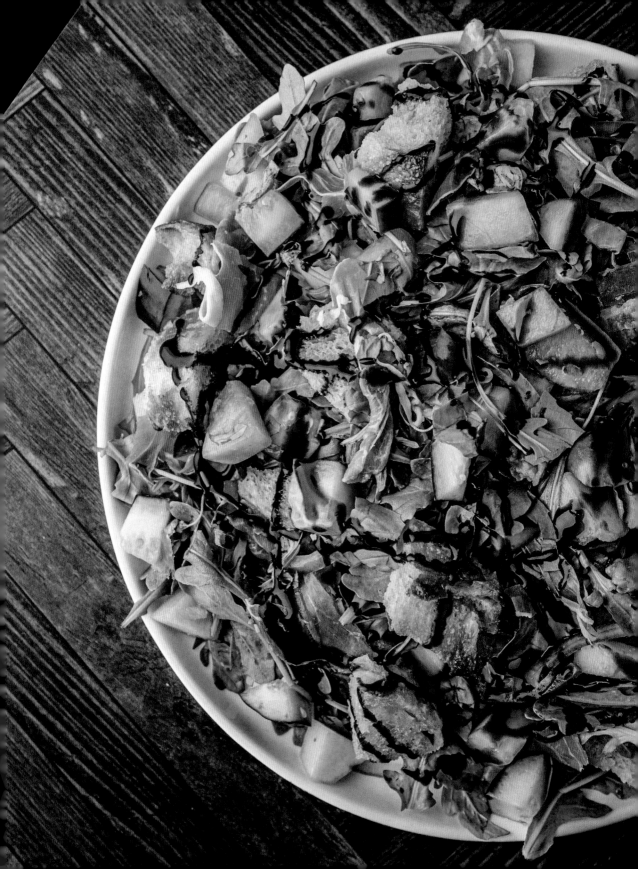

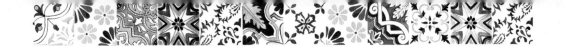

Melon and Prosciutto
PANZANELLA

SERVES 6 Prep time: 15 minutes ✳ Cook time: 10 minutes

We love a classic Italian panzanella, the simple tomato, onion, and bread salad. But we equally adore riffing on the recipe just as Italian people do, and we have done a variation in almost every cookbook! When Deanna enjoyed a cantaloupe panzanella at a local Italian restaurant, she knew we had to recreate it for this book. Cantaloupe is rich in beta-carotene—which is potentially linked to reducing depression—among other vitamins and minerals tied to positive cognitive health.

½ red onion, thinly sliced

¼ cup orange juice

4 cups cubed sourdough or other crusty bread (½-inch pieces—see Hack)

3 tablespoons extra-virgin olive oil

2 cups chopped cantaloupe (½-inch pieces)

1 large cucumber, chopped into ½-inch pieces (about 2 cups)

2 cups arugula

½ cup finely chopped fresh basil leaves and stems

3 ounces prosciutto, sliced into 2-inch pieces

¼ teaspoon black pepper

2 tablespoons balsamic vinegar

Preheat the oven to 425°F.

Put the sliced onion in a shallow bowl. Pour in the orange juice so it's covering all the pieces. (This step helps tame the pungency of the onion.) Set aside as you toast the bread.

Put the bread pieces on a large rimmed baking sheet and drizzle with the oil. Using your hands, toss until the bread is well coated, then spread out on the sheet. Bake for 10 to 12 minutes, until the edges are crispy. Transfer to a large serving bowl. Add the onion with the juice, cantaloupe, cucumber, arugula, basil, prosciutto, and pepper. Gently toss together. Right before serving, drizzle with the balsamic vinegar, toss again, and serve.

Healthy Kitchen Hack: We purposely called this "Melon" Panzanella to encourage you to try different melons like honeydew or watermelon in place of the cantaloupe. Or get adventurous during stone fruit season and swap in chopped peaches, nectarines, plums, and/or apricots for the melon. And while we think it's worth taking the 10 minutes to make the olive oil–infused "croutons," you can skip the cooking step by using stale bread and then tossing the finished salad with the olive oil.

PER SERVING: Calories: 258; Total Fat: 10g; Saturated Fat: 2g; Cholesterol: 3mg; Sodium: 564mg; Total Carbohydrates: 34g; Fiber: 2g; Protein: 10g

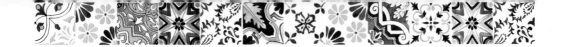

Green Couscous
LETTUCE SCOOPS

SERVES 6 Prep time: 20 minutes ✳ Cook time: 5 minutes

1 cup couscous
(not Israeli couscous)

¼ teaspoon kosher
or sea salt

1½ cups frozen peas,
thawed (see Hack)

1 lemon

1 recipe Speedy Pesto
Sauce (page 130)

1 head iceberg lettuce
or 2 heads butter lettuce

1 teaspoon extra-virgin
olive oil

¼ teaspoon black pepper

This is one of our "looks fancy but is easy to make" recipes, so you don't have to save these attractive lettuce cups for guests. While creating this dish, Serena discovered they're perfect for helping salad-avoiding kids (and adults) eat more greens. Antioxidant-rich leafy greens and herbs are excellent for brain health, and so are all the healthy fats found in the fluffy couscous stuffing, including olive oil and nuts/seeds in the pesto.

Bring 1½ cups water to a boil in a medium saucepan. Stir in the couscous and salt and cover. Remove from the heat and let stand for 5 minutes, then stir in the peas and fluff with a fork; set aside.

While the couscous heats, using a Microplane or citrus zester, grate the zest from the lemon into a large bowl, then cut the lemon in half and squeeze in the juice from one half. Cut the remaining half into wedges for serving. Add the cooked couscous with peas and toss with the lemon juice to combine; cool to room temperature, then stir in the pesto.

To assemble, separate the lettuce into six "cups" of 2 to 3 leaves stacked atop each other, and arrange on a serving platter. Top each "cup" with about ½ cup of the couscous mixture. Drizzle the platter with the oil and top with the black pepper. Serve with the lemon wedges for squeezing.

PER SERVING: Calories: 299; Total Fat: 15g; Saturated Fat: 3g; Cholesterol: 4mg; Sodium: 200mg; Total Carbohydrates: 34g; Fiber: 6g; Protein: 9g

Healthy Kitchen Hack: Frozen peas are perfectly yummy...as long as you don't overcook them. We always have a bag in the freezer and toss them into soups, pasta dishes, scrambled eggs, and even Greek yogurt with a sprinkle of sea salt and a drizzle of olive oil. To thaw, simply pour the peas into a bowl on the counter as you prep a recipe or meal. Or, if pasta is on the menu, toss the peas into the colander and drain the pasta over the peas.

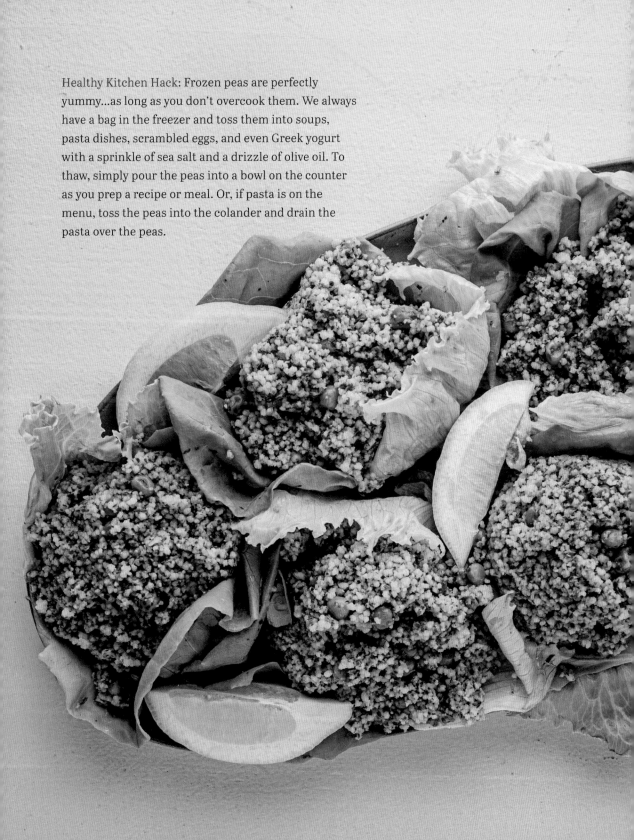

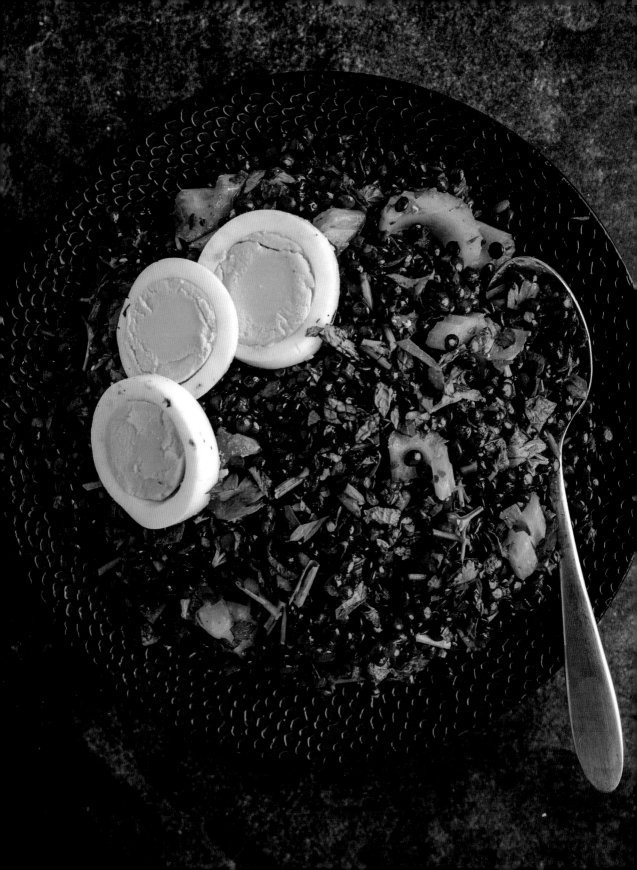

BLACK LENTIL SALAD
with Toasted Cumin

SERVES 6   Prep time: 10 minutes   ❋   Cook time: 30 minutes

Expand your lentil horizons and try black lentils in this simple yet zesty salad. Tiny in shape and a bit peppery in flavor, black lentils look striking in this dish, especially with the bright pops of green herbs and contrasting white and yellow of sliced hard-boiled eggs. The zestiness comes from cumin seeds, which are traditional to cuisines around the Mediterranean, and because they're whole seeds, they add a pinch of antioxidants. When toasted, the spice delivers earthy, slightly sweet flavors with an edge of citrus to this salad, to any pot of whole grains, or to a homemade vinaigrette dressing.

Heat 2 tablespoons oil in a large saucepan or Dutch oven over medium heat. Add the garlic, cumin, and pepper and cook, stirring occasionally until fragrant, 1 minute. Add the lentils, ½ teaspoon salt, and 2½ cups water and bring to a boil over high heat. Reduce the heat to medium-low, partially cover to vent, and simmer for 25 to 30 minutes, until the lentils are tender but not mushy; they should still have a slight firmness to them.

While the lentils cook, using a Microplane or citrus zester, grate the zest from the lemon into a large bowl, then cut the lemon in half and squeeze in the juice. Whisk in the remaining 1 tablespoon oil and remaining ½ teaspoon salt. Stir in the celery.

continued on page 76

3 tablespoons extra-virgin olive oil, divided

2 garlic cloves, sliced

½ teaspoon cumin seeds or 1 teaspoon ground cumin

¼ teaspoon Aleppo chile flakes or crushed red pepper

1 cup black or brown lentils

1 teaspoon kosher or sea salt, divided

1 lemon

2 celery ribs with leaves, sliced diagonally

1 cup chopped fresh cilantro leaves and stems

½ cup chopped fresh mint leaves

2 hard-boiled large eggs (see Hack), sliced

continued from page 75

Add the cooked lentils to the bowl and stir to combine with the dressing. Let the salad cool for 5 minutes for the flavors to meld. Stir in the cilantro and mint. Transfer the lentil salad to a serving platter and top with the eggs. Serve warm, at room temperature, or chilled.

Healthy Kitchen Hack: We never pass up a chance to "put an egg on it" because of eggs' stellar nutrient profile and the overall enhancement they bring to any recipe. For perfect hard-boiled eggs, put 4 to 6 large eggs in a saucepan and cover with water by 1 inch. Bring to a boil, then cover, remove from the burner, and let sit covered for 13 minutes. Immediately transfer the eggs to a large bowl of ice water to cool completely for easier shelling.

66
We liked the texture and the taste of black lentils and how they cooked quickly.

BECKY FROM
PORTLAND, ME

PER SERVING: Calories: 207; Total Fat: 9g; Saturated Fat: 2g; Cholesterol: 62mg; Sodium: 248mg; Total Carbohydrates: 22g; Fiber: 4g; Protein: 10g

Spicy GREEN BEAN AND POTATO SALAD

SERVES 6   Prep time: 15 minutes   ❋   Cook time: 10 minutes

A little bit of spicy kick in many of our recipes makes the food tastier and more balanced, but without adding too much heat. Our twist on the potato salad is a textbook example: tender potatoes, firm green beans, and crunchy seeds, tossed with tart vinegar, tingly chilies, cumin, herbs, and buttery olive oil. Every ingredient—especially those spicy chilies (see the Hack)—is good for our brains.

In a small bowl, whisk together the vinegar, garlic, cumin, chile flakes, salt, and black pepper. Set aside to allow the garlic to mellow.

Put the potatoes in a large saucepan. Cover the potatoes with water by 1 inch. Bring to a boil. Reduce the heat to medium-low and cook for 6 to 8 minutes, until fork-tender. Using a slotted spoon, skimmer, or kitchen spider, carefully transfer the potatoes to a serving bowl. Bring the water to a boil again. Add the beans to the water and boil for 1 to 2 minutes, until bright green. Using the slotted spoon, transfer the beans to the bowl with the potatoes.

Whisk the oil into the vinegar mixture. Pour the dressing over the salad and gently toss to combine. Add the cilantro and seeds and toss to combine. Serve warm or cold.

Healthy Kitchen Hack: Try all the chile peppers the Mediterranean has to offer (See page 15) in some of these ways:

▸ Sprinkle the raisiny, almost sweet Urfa into cottage cheese, plain yogurt with honey, or chocolate desserts.

▸ Add the mildly spicy Aleppo to fruit salads, green salads, or anything with lots of fresh green herbs.

▸ Mix a pinch of smoked paprika into any egg or bean dish.

1 tablespoon red or white wine vinegar

1 garlic clove, minced

½ teaspoon cumin seeds or ground cumin

¼–½ teaspoon Urfa or Aleppo chile flakes or crushed red pepper

¼ teaspoon kosher or sea salt

¼ teaspoon black pepper

1½ pounds small red or yellow potatoes, quartered

8 ounces green beans, trimmed

3 tablespoons extra-virgin olive oil

1 cup chopped fresh cilantro and/or parsley leaves and stems

¼ cup sunflower seeds, pepitas, pistachios, chopped walnuts, and/or other nuts or seeds

PER SERVING:
Calories: 208; Total Fat: 10g; Saturated Fat: 1g; Cholesterol: 0mg; Sodium: 104mg; Total Carbohydrates: 27g; Fiber: 4g; Protein: 4g

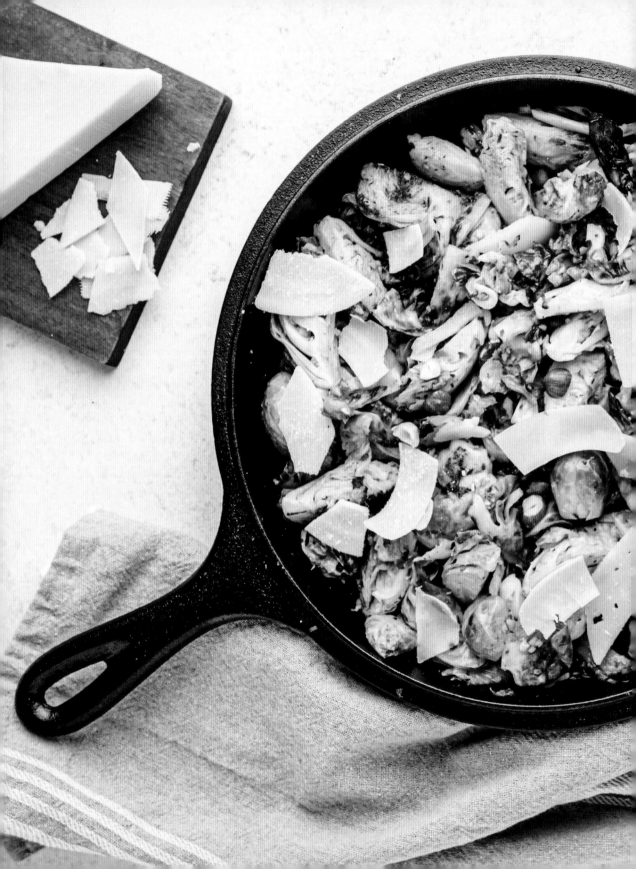

SIDES

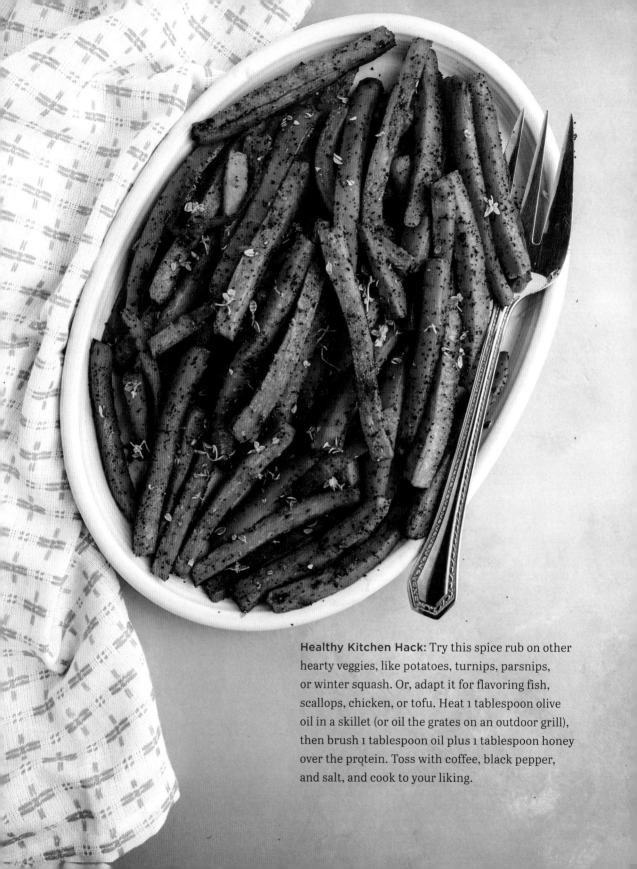

Healthy Kitchen Hack: Try this spice rub on other hearty veggies, like potatoes, turnips, parsnips, or winter squash. Or, adapt it for flavoring fish, scallops, chicken, or tofu. Heat 1 tablespoon olive oil in a skillet (or oil the grates on an outdoor grill), then brush 1 tablespoon oil plus 1 tablespoon honey over the protein. Toss with coffee, black pepper, and salt, and cook to your liking.

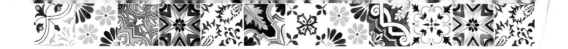

Black Pepper and Coffee
ROASTED CARROTS

SERVES 8 Prep time: 10 minutes ☀ Cook time: 30 minutes

It might sound like an unlikely combo, but the powerful flavors of honey, coffee, and black pepper will make your roasted carrots irresistible. While this recipe uses a smaller amount of ground coffee compared to a brewed cup, moderate doses of caffeine from coffee beans can help counter feelings of depression and may even lift one's mood. Paired with black pepper, those coffee beans supercharge this side dish with brain benefits.

Arrange the oven racks in the upper-middle and lower-middle positions. Preheat the oven to 450°F. Coat two large rimmed baking sheets with cooking spray.

Cut the carrots in half lengthwise and cut each half into 3-inch sticks, so all the pieces are roughly the same thickness (if a piece is too thick, cut it in half lengthwise again). Put the carrots in a large bowl. Drizzle with the oil and 4 teaspoons honey and, using your hands, toss well. Sprinkle with the coffee, black pepper, and salt and toss again until well coated.

Spread out the carrots evenly on the baking sheets and drizzle with any remaining coffee glaze in the bowl. Roast for 15 minutes, remove the sheets from the oven, and stir. Return the sheets to the opposite racks and roast for an additional 10 to 15 minutes, until the carrots are very tender with a few crispy ends. Transfer the carrots to a serving dish and sprinkle with the thyme. Drizzle with the remaining 2 teaspoons honey and top with the orange or lemon zest. Serve with additional thyme on top, if desired.

Tip: To make these carrots vegan, swap in brown sugar for the 4 teaspoons honey added before roasting and skip the final honey drizzle step.

2 pounds carrots, trimmed and scrubbed

2 tablespoons extra-virgin olive oil

6 teaspoons honey, divided

1 tablespoon finely ground coffee beans (unbrewed)

1¼ teaspoons black pepper

¼ teaspoon kosher or sea salt

1 tablespoon fresh thyme leaves or 1 teaspoon dried thyme, plus more for garnish (optional)

Grated zest of 1 orange or lemon

66

I'm a coffee lover, so these roasted carrots were a hit!

SIMON FROM
HULL, MA

PER SERVING:
Calories: 95; Total Fat: 4g;
Saturated Fat: 1g;
Cholesterol: 0mg;
Sodium: 139mg;
Total Carbohydrates: 16g;
Fiber: 3g; Protein: 1g

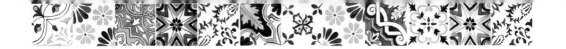

Magical OLIVE OIL POTATO HASH

SERVES 6   Prep time: 10 minutes ✻ Cook time: 30 minutes

4 tablespoons extra-virgin olive oil, divided

1 pound Italian eggplant (about 1 medium) or zucchini (about 2 medium), trimmed and cut into ¾-inch cubes, or 1 pound green beans

1 teaspoon kosher or sea salt, divided

1½ pounds gold or red potatoes (about 4 medium), unpeeled

2 tablespoons red wine vinegar

1 tablespoon tomato paste

2 garlic cloves, chopped

2–3 tablespoons chopped fresh dill

Not surprisingly, we go through many bottles and tins of extra-virgin olive oil. As the prominent cooking staple of Mediterranean cuisine, it is largely responsible for many of the health benefits associated with the Mediterranean Diet, including helping with short-term memory and decreasing dementia risk. But it's olive oil's buttery, peppery properties that make veggies go from "meh" to magical. If you aren't fond of eggplant (or zucchini or green beans), try slow-cooking in several tablespoons of olive oil, as we do here, which results in a silky and lusciously flavored version of the veggie.

In a large cast-iron or nonstick skillet, heat 3 tablespoons oil over medium heat. Distribute the eggplant evenly in the pan. Sprinkle with ½ teaspoon salt. Cook (without stirring) until the eggplant begins to brown, about 5 minutes. Continue to cook, stirring occasionally, until very soft, 10 to 12 additional minutes. Transfer the cooked eggplant to a plate.

While the eggplant cooks, shred the potatoes on the large holes of a box grater. Wrap them in a clean towel and squeeze out the moisture. Transfer the potatoes to a paper towel–lined plate and microwave on high for 2 minutes (this step yields better browning potatoes).

Add the remaining 1 tablespoon olive oil to the skillet. When the oil is very hot, distribute the potatoes evenly in the pan. Sprinkle with the remaining ½ teaspoon salt and cook (without stirring) until the potatoes begin to brown, about 5 minutes. Continue to cook, stirring occasionally, until the potatoes are golden, 2 to 4 additional minutes.

Meanwhile, in a small bowl, whisk together 3 tablespoons water, the vinegar, tomato paste, and garlic. Set aside.

When the potatoes are done, return the eggplant to the skillet and stir to combine. Push the vegetables to the outer edges of the skillet and add the vinegar mixture. Stir, scraping up the brown bits on the bottom of the skillet until the garlic is soft, about 3 more minutes, then stir in the vegetables from the sides until the vinegar mixture is incorporated into the vegetables. Remove the skillet from the heat, top with the fresh dill, and serve.

Tip: This recipe is not crispy hash browns, but more like the moister New England-style potato hash.

Healthy Kitchen Hack: One of our favorite convenience foods is frozen shredded hash brown potatoes. They are zero-food waste because there's no prep and the only ingredient is potatoes (and sometimes a simple preservative to keep them from turning brown). Use them in place of freshly shredded potatoes in just about any recipe. The cooking times and directions will be the same because even though they need a little time to thaw in the skillet, they actually cook a bit faster than fresh.

66

I usually make crispy hash browns, but this hash has a softer texture, which I also like because the sauce is so good. And the olive oil really does make the eggplant magically creamy.

GLORIA FROM
LOS ANGELES, CA

PER SERVING: Calories: 186, Total Fat: 10g; Saturated Fat: 1g; Cholesterol: 0mg; Sodium: 342mg; Total Carbohydrates: 24g; Fiber: 6g; Protein: 3g

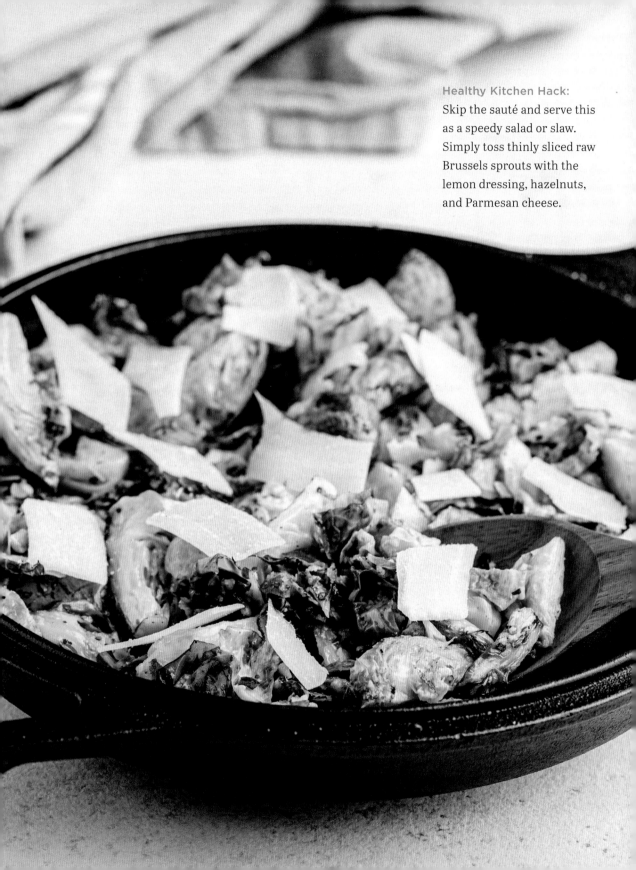

Healthy Kitchen Hack:
Skip the sauté and serve this as a speedy salad or slaw. Simply toss thinly sliced raw Brussels sprouts with the lemon dressing, hazelnuts, and Parmesan cheese.

BRUSSELS SPROUT SAUTÉ
with Hazelnuts

SERVES 6 Prep time: 10 minutes ✳ Cook time: 10 minutes

Our fabulous dietetic intern, Kevin, recreated his all-time favorite item from Trader Joe's grocery store, the Brussels Sprout Sauté Kit. This quick pan-cooked side is a savory and smart choice to make come fall and winter. Brussels sprouts are a top source of vitamin K, which may be helpful for people at risk for dementia and may also help reduce depression, anxiety, and cognitive impairment. Olive oil helps our bodies absorb the fat-soluble vitamin K, plus it makes brussels sprouts super palatable.

1 lemon

6 tablespoons extra-virgin olive oil, divided

1 garlic clove, minced

1 teaspoon Dijon mustard

¼ teaspoon kosher or sea salt

¼ teaspoon black pepper

1 pound brussels sprouts, quartered or sliced ¼ inch thick

⅓ cup chopped hazelnuts

⅓ cup shaved Parmesan or Pecorino Romano cheese (about 1 ounce)

Using a Microplane or citrus zester, grate the zest from the lemon into a wide-mouthed jar with a lid (or a bowl), then cut the lemon in half and squeeze in the juice from half of the lemon (save the remaining lemon half for another use). To the jar, add 4 tablespoons oil, the garlic, mustard, salt, and pepper. Close the lid tightly and shake to mix (or whisk the dressing in a bowl). Set aside.

Heat the remaining 2 tablespoons oil in a large skillet over medium-high heat. Add the brussels sprouts and cook for 4 minutes, stirring only after a few become browned but are still tender-crisp. Add the hazelnuts and cook for 2 minutes, until they start to smell toasted, stirring occasionally. Add the lemon dressing and cook for another 2 minutes, until the sprouts are a little more tender but still crisp. Sprinkle with the cheese and serve warm.

PER SERVING: Calories: 215; Total Fat: 19g; Saturated Fat: 3g; Cholesterol: 3mg; Sodium: 201mg; Total Carbohydrates: 9g; Fiber: 4g; Protein: 5g

PAN-ROASTED MUSHROOMS
in Wine and Thyme

SERVES 4 Prep time: 10 minutes ✳ Cook time: 25 minutes

3 tablespoons extra-virgin olive oil, divided

2 pounds mushrooms (any kind), sliced

2 garlic cloves, minced

3 tablespoons fresh thyme leaves, divided

¼ teaspoon kosher or sea salt

¼ teaspoon black pepper

⅓ cup dry red wine

1 tablespoon balsamic vinegar

Meet your brain's best friend—the humble mushroom! Eco-friendly to grow and delivering a savory, meaty flavor, mushrooms are one of the few natural sources of vitamin D. This vitamin, plus specific antioxidants found in mushrooms, may explain why they've been tied to reducing risk for depression. So, when you are stumped on what side to make for dinner, strive to make mushrooms more often!

In a large skillet, heat 1 tablespoon oil over medium-high heat. Add half of the mushrooms, mix to coat, and then cook, stirring occasionally, until most of the liquid has cooked off, 8 to 10 minutes. Transfer the mushrooms to a serving bowl. Heat another 1 tablespoon oil in the skillet. Stir in the remaining mushrooms and cook as with the first batch. Transfer to the bowl.

Reduce the heat to medium and heat the remaining 1 tablespoon olive oil. Add the garlic, 2 tablespoons thyme, salt, and pepper and cook, stirring constantly (to avoid burning the garlic), for 30 seconds. Return all the mushrooms to the skillet and mix until well coated. Pour in the wine and vinegar and cook, stirring occasionally, for 3 to 5 minutes, until the sauce thickens to your liking. Sprinkle with the remaining 1 tablespoon thyme and serve warm.

Tip: Serve these with our Steak au Poivre (page 204) or Crispy Za'atar Tilapia with Orange Slices (page 191), or over your favorite pasta or whole grain.

Healthy Kitchen Hack:
Mushrooms are super adaptable when it comes to spicing or "herbing" them up. Add rosemary and/ or parsley to the thyme in this recipe. Try tarragon or sage. Or spice them up with smoked paprika, za'atar, everything bagel seasoning, chile flakes, or extra garlic.

PER SERVING: Calories: 163; Total Fat: 11g; Saturated Fat: 2g; Cholesterol: 0mg; Sodium: 133mg; Total Carbohydrates: 10g; Fiber: 3g; Protein: 7g

CORN, CILANTRO, AND POMEGRANATE *Medley*

SERVES 6 Prep time: 15 minutes

When you want an upgrade from a basic potato salad or slaw side, this gorgeous veggie dish is your answer. Make it during pomegranate season (typically from September to December in North America), when you can find them in the store or farmers' market, if you're lucky enough to live in a climate where they grow freely. This side is studded with plant-based nutrients and colorful antioxidants that come into play for better brain and mental health. But most memorable are the colors, textures, and layered flavors of this easy veggie side—we're sure everyone will be asking you for the recipe!

1 (16-ounce) bag frozen corn, thawed (see Hack)

1 avocado, peeled, pitted, and diced

1 cup pomegranate arils (seeds)

½ red onion, diced

½ teaspoon ground cumin

½ teaspoon smoked paprika

½ teaspoon kosher or sea salt, divided

3 tablespoons extra-virgin olive oil

2 tablespoons balsamic vinegar

1 tablespoon orange juice

1 tablespoon honey

¼ teaspoon black pepper

1 cup chopped fresh cilantro leaves and stems

In a large serving bowl, mix the corn, avocado, pomegranate arils, onion, cumin, smoked paprika, and ¼ teaspoon salt. Set aside.

To make the dressing, in a small bowl, whisk together the oil, vinegar, orange juice, honey, pepper, and remaining ¼ teaspoon salt.

Right before serving, mix the cilantro into the corn medley. Pour in the dressing and toss gently until all ingredients are coated.

Healthy Kitchen Hack: If you live in a climate where corn and pomegranate seasons overlap (we are envious!), swap in the kernels from 4 cooked ears of corn for the frozen corn. Or use 2 (14-ounce) cans corn, drained, instead. For another layer of flavor, look for fire-roasted canned or frozen corn varieties.

PER SERVING: Calories: 198; Total Fat: 11g; Saturated Fat: 2g; Cholesterol: 0mg; Sodium: 169mg; Total Carbohydrates: 26g; Fiber: 5g; Protein: 3g

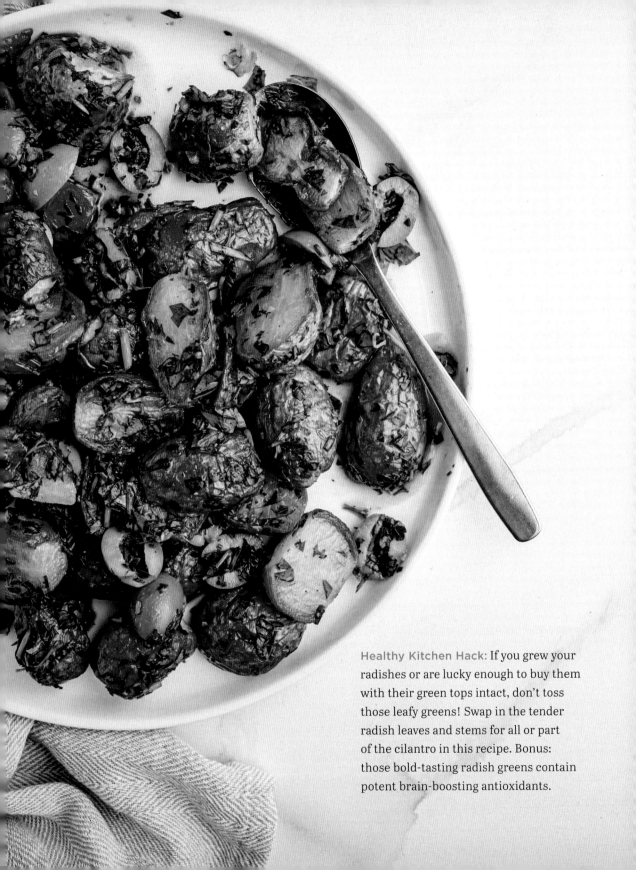

Healthy Kitchen Hack: If you grew your radishes or are lucky enough to buy them with their green tops intact, don't toss those leafy greens! Swap in the tender radish leaves and stems for all or part of the cilantro in this recipe. Bonus: those bold-tasting radish greens contain potent brain-boosting antioxidants.

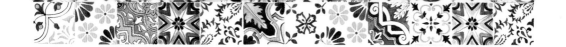

ROASTED RADISHES
with Green Olive Salsa Verde

SERVES 6 Prep time: 15 minutes ✳ Cook time: 20 minutes

When it comes to vegetable gardening, the humble radish is pretty close to instant gratification. About three weeks after planting radish seeds, you can have a bountiful harvest. Growing your own radishes means added brain benefits, too: eliminating the travel time from farm to store means fewer nutrients are lost in transportation. Of course, raw radishes are delectable with their sharp, refreshing flavor, but when roasted, they take on a sweet, peppery taste that pairs perfectly with this bright green, buttery, lemony relish.

1¼ pounds radishes, halved

3 tablespoons extra-virgin olive oil, divided

¼ teaspoon kosher or sea salt

5 garlic cloves, unpeeled and lightly smashed

1 lemon

½ cup chopped green olives plus ¼ cup olive liquid, divided

¼ teaspoon black pepper

¼ teaspoon crushed red pepper

1½ cups chopped fresh cilantro leaves and stems

Preheat the oven to 400°F.

Put the radishes on a large rimmed baking sheet, drizzle with 1 tablespoon oil, and sprinkle with the salt. Toss to coat, then arrange cut side down. Place the smashed garlic cloves on a 6 × 6-inch piece of aluminum foil and drizzle with ½ tablespoon oil. Fold the foil into a packet around the garlic and place it on the baking sheet. Roast for about 20 minutes, until the radishes are tender and the garlic is very soft. Unwrap the garlic to cool slightly.

When cool enough to handle, remove the garlic skins and transfer the warm garlic and any oil remaining from the packet into a large bowl. Using a fork, mash into a chunky paste. Using a Microplane or citrus zester, grate the zest from the lemon over the garlic, then cut the lemon in half and squeeze in the juice from half of the lemon (save the remaining lemon half for another use). Whisk in the remaining 1½ tablespoons oil, olive liquid, black pepper, and red pepper. Stir in the olives and cilantro. Add the warm or room-temperature radishes and toss to combine and serve.

PER SERVING:
Calories: 97; Total Fat: 8g;
Saturated Fat: 1g;
Cholesterol: 0mg;
Sodium: 348mg;
Total Carbohydrates: 6g;
Fiber: 2g; Protein: 1g

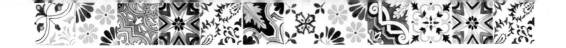

SAUTÉED GREENS
with Honey-Tahini Sauce

SERVES 4   Prep time: 15 minutes ✳ Cook time: 20 minutes

1 bunch hardy dark greens (such as collards, kale, mustard greens, or Swiss chard)

3 tablespoons extra-virgin olive oil, divided

3 garlic cloves, minced

1 teaspoon ground cumin

¼ teaspoon kosher or sea salt

¼ teaspoon black pepper

1 lemon

2 tablespoons tahini

2 teaspoons honey

1 tablespoon sesame seeds (optional)

Let's face it, dark leafy greens aren't everyone's favorite veggies. But this irresistible zesty sauce—whipped up in seconds with honey, tahini, lemon juice, and olive oil—can take collards from "meh" to "yeah"! And it's probably not surprising that these greens are abundant in nutrients that protect our brains, strengthen cognitive awareness, and improve mental health.

Lay 3 or 4 greens leaves on top of each other and fold in half so the stem is at the fold. Run your knife down the inside of the thick stems, removing them from the leaves. Repeat with the remaining leaves. Chop the stems into ¼-inch pieces. Chop the leaves into ½-inch slices, keeping them separate from the chopped stems. You'll have 7 to 8 cups chopped greens.

In a large stockpot, heat 2 tablespoons olive oil over medium heat. Add the chopped stems and cook, stirring occasionally, until slightly softened, about 3 minutes. Add the garlic and cook, stirring frequently, for 30 seconds. Add the chopped green leaves, cumin, salt, pepper, and ¼ cup water, then stir well to coat. Using a Microplane or citrus zester, grate the zest from the lemon into the pot, then cut the lemon in half and squeeze in the juice from one half (reserve the other half for the tahini sauce). Stir all the ingredients, then reduce the heat to medium-low, cover, and cook, stirring twice, until the greens soften, about 15 minutes. Remove from the heat and let cool for 5 to 10 minutes.

While the greens cool, make the tahini sauce. Squeeze the juice from the remaining lemon half into a small bowl. Add the tahini, honey, and remaining 1 tablespoon oil. As you

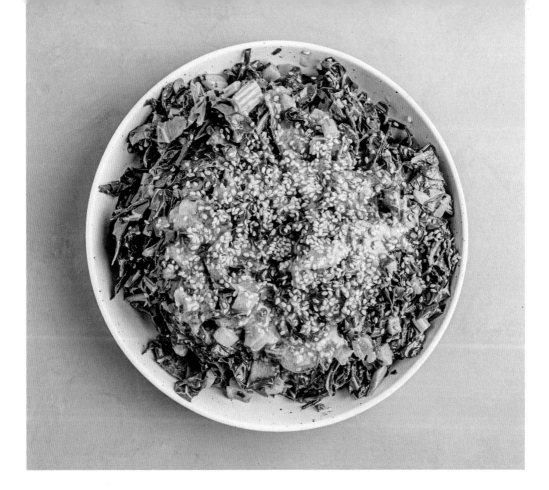

whisk the ingredients together, add 1 tablespoon cold water and continue to whisk until a pourable sauce forms.

To serve, spoon the greens onto each plate. Drizzle with the honey-tahini sauce and sprinkle with sesame seeds, if desired.

Tip: You can swap in delicate greens like spinach or arugula, but shorten the cooking time by about 10 minutes.

Healthy Kitchen Hack: Confession: Deanna had to make extra honey tahini sauce while trying out this recipe as she found herself taste testing it a little too much—it's that good. Make a double batch and try it drizzled over roasted vegetables, tossed with salad greens, swirled into yogurt, spread on toast, or smeared on your favorite sandwich. (Deanna loves it paired with grilled cheese.)

PER SERVING: Calories: 189; Total Fat: 16g; Saturated Fat: 2g; Cholesterol: 0mg; Sodium: 137mg; Total Carbohydrates: 11g; Fiber: 4g; Protein: 4g

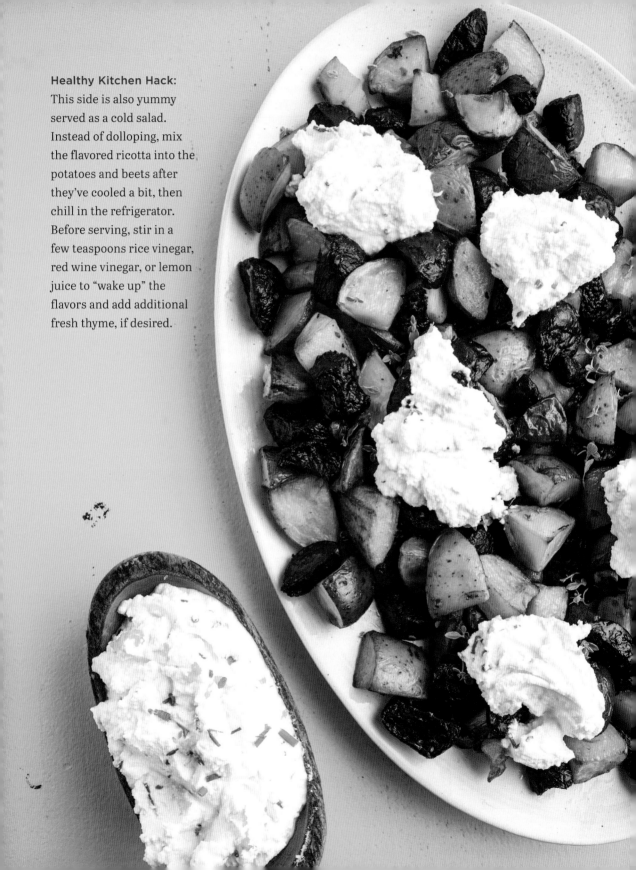

Healthy Kitchen Hack:
This side is also yummy
served as a cold salad.
Instead of dolloping, mix
the flavored ricotta into the
potatoes and beets after
they've cooled a bit, then
chill in the refrigerator.
Before serving, stir in a
few teaspoons rice vinegar,
red wine vinegar, or lemon
juice to "wake up" the
flavors and add additional
fresh thyme, if desired.

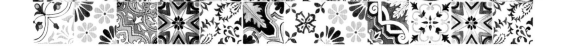

ROASTED POTATOES AND BEETS *with Herbed Ricotta*

SERVES 8   Prep time: 10 minutes   ✳   Cook time: 35 minutes

For the beet avoiders out there, please try this recipe before you swear off beets for good! Here we pair the red and golden root veggie with the loveable potato, roast them both to perfection, then cool them off with an Italian-inspired flavored ricotta "topping." New research suggests that beets may help delay memory decline by improving blood flow to the brain—yet another reason to embrace them into your veggie routine.

Arrange the oven racks in the upper-middle and lower-middle positions. Preheat the oven to 425°F. Coat two large rimmed baking sheets with cooking spray.

In a large bowl, combine the potatoes, beets, olive oil, the leaves from 5 thyme sprigs, salt, and pepper. Toss until the vegetables are well coated. Spread out evenly on the baking sheets. Roast for 15 minutes, remove the sheets from the oven, add the garlic, and stir. Return the sheets to the opposite racks and roast for an additional 15 to 20 minutes, until the vegetables are fork-tender and the potatoes start to crisp. Transfer to a serving platter and sprinkle with the remaining thyme leaves.

While the vegetables cook, put the ricotta, chives, and orange zest in a small serving bowl and mix.

To serve, dollop about half of the ricotta mix in spoonfuls on top of the roasted potatoes and beets, then garnish with extra thyme, if desired. Serve with the remaining ricotta on the side.

2 pounds baby, red, and/or Yukon Gold potatoes, scrubbed and cut into 1-inch pieces

2 pounds red and/or golden beets, scrubbed and cut into 1-inch pieces

3 tablespoons extra-virgin olive oil

Leaves from 10 thyme sprigs, divided, plus more for garnish (optional)

¼ teaspoon kosher or sea salt

¼ teaspoon black pepper

3 garlic cloves, thinly sliced

1 (15-ounce) container whole-milk ricotta

1 tablespoon chopped fresh chives

1 teaspoon grated orange zest

66

This recipe got me to try beets, and they were delicious roasted in this dish.

JANE FROM
SUDBURY, MA

PER SERVING: Calories: 269; Total Fat: 13g; Saturated Fat: 5g; Cholesterol: 28mg; Sodium: 212mg; Total Carbohydrates: 31g; Fiber: 6g; Protein: 10g

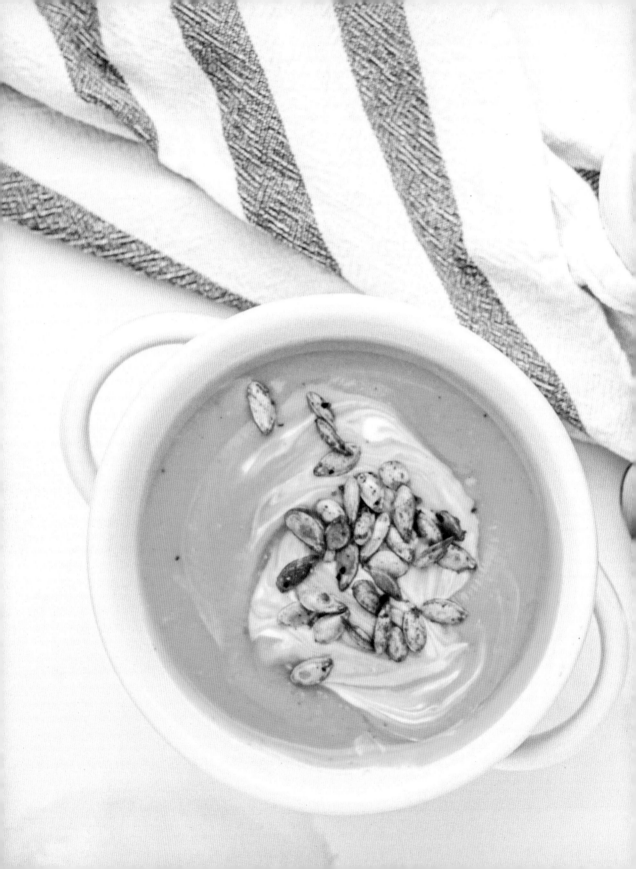

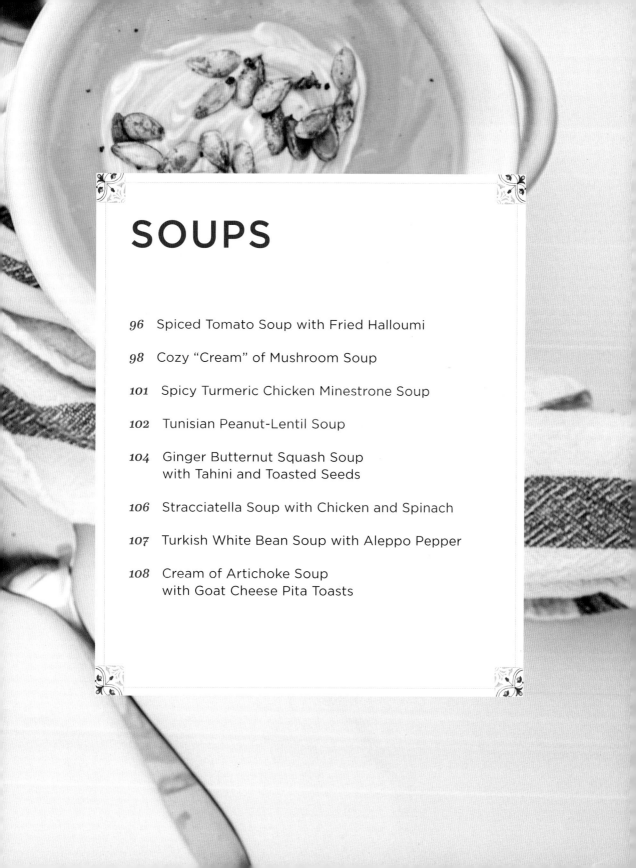

SOUPS

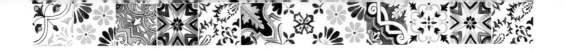

SPICED TOMATO SOUP
with Fried Halloumi

SERVES 6 Prep time: 10 minutes ❋ Cook time: 20 minutes

1 tablespoon plus
2 teaspoons extra-virgin
olive oil, divided

1 onion, diced

1 carrot, scrubbed
and shredded

¼ cup dry red wine
or 1 tablespoon
red wine vinegar plus
3 tablespoons water

2 teaspoons
dried oregano,
plus more for garnish

¾ teaspoon
ground cinnamon

½ teaspoon black pepper

1 (28-ounce) can
low-sodium crushed
tomatoes

1 (14.5-ounce) can
low-sodium diced
tomatoes, undrained

8 ounces halloumi cheese,
cut into ½-inch-thick slices
(see Hack for substitute)

Spoon up tomato soup with grilled cheese the Mediterranean way! Halloumi cheese is pan-fried into golden melty squares to dunk in comforting bowls of cinnamon and black pepper spiced tomato soup. Cinnamon is common in many savory dishes around the Mediterranean, including in Greece, where it's prized for the warmth and slight earthiness that it adds to dishes like beef kapama stew, rice and tomato recipes, and pastitsio (this soup is the base sauce for our Mushroom Pastitsio "Baked" Pasta on page 148). Cinnamon is also prized for its many brain benefits, including potentially helping to delay cognitive impairment.

Heat 1 tablespoon oil in a large pot or Dutch oven over medium heat. Add the onion and carrot and cook, stirring occasionally, until they soften, 8 to 10 minutes. Add the red wine, oregano, cinnamon, and pepper and cook, stirring occasionally, until the liquid evaporates, about 2 minutes. Add the tomatoes with their juices and 1½ cups water (use the water to rinse the diced tomato can) and add to the pot. Cook, stirring occasionally until the soup boils. Turn the heat to low and simmer for 5 minutes for the flavors to meld.

While the soup simmers, heat the remaining 2 teaspoons oil in a large skillet over medium-high heat. When the oil is very hot, add the halloumi slices. Cook until golden, 1 to 2 minutes, flip the slices, and cook until golden on the other side, about 1 minute. Transfer the cheese to a paper towel–lined plate. Immediately pour the soup into four bowls. Cut the halloumi into squares and distribute evenly on top of each bowl. Sprinkle the bowls with extra oregano.

PER SERVING: Calories: 267; Total Fat: 16g; Saturated Fat: 9g; Cholesterol: 33mg; Sodium: 602mg; Total Carbohydrates: 17g; Fiber: 4g; Protein: 13g

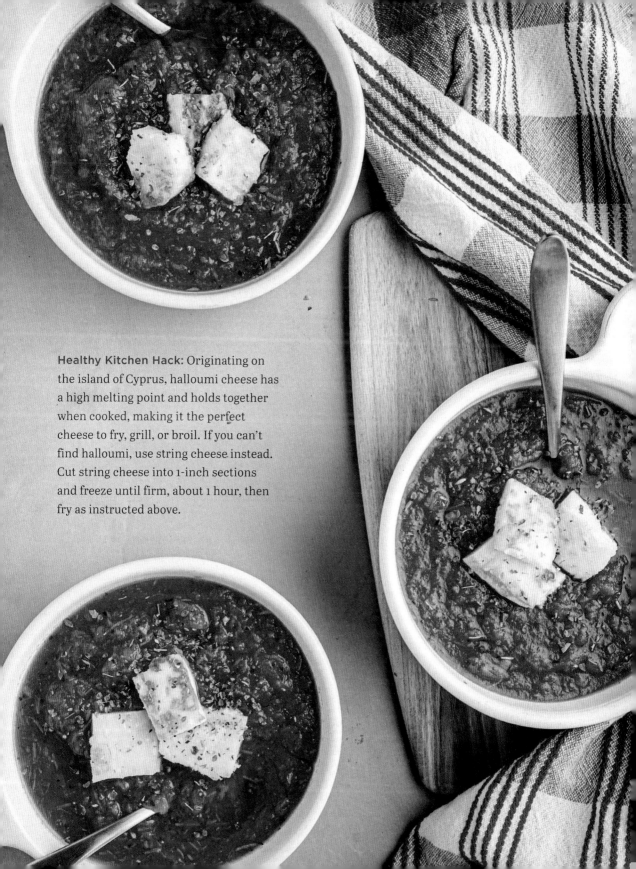

Healthy Kitchen Hack: Originating on the island of Cyprus, halloumi cheese has a high melting point and holds together when cooked, making it the perfect cheese to fry, grill, or broil. If you can't find halloumi, use string cheese instead. Cut string cheese into 1-inch sections and freeze until firm, about 1 hour, then fry as instructed above.

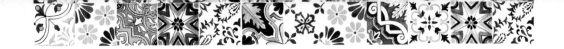

Cozy "CREAM" OF MUSHROOM SOUP

SERVES 6   Prep time: 10 minutes ✳ Cook time: 30 minutes

2 tablespoons extra-virgin olive oil

2 celery ribs, diced

1 onion, diced

1 pound mushrooms (such as button, cremini, and/or others), sliced

2 teaspoons sweet paprika

½ teaspoon smoked paprika

¼ teaspoon kosher or sea salt

¼ teaspoon black pepper

1 large russet potato, scrubbed and cut into ½-inch cubes

2 tablespoons all-purpose flour

3 cups low-sodium vegetable broth

1 bay leaf

1 cup plain whole-milk Greek yogurt or Homemade Yogurt (page 60), divided

1 tablespoon red or white wine vinegar

¼ cup chopped fresh dill or parsley leaves

From truffles and cèpes (porcini) in the South of France to morels and vrganj (another version of porcini) in Croatia, mushrooms grow throughout the Mediterranean and are showcased in many traditional dishes. This recipe, featuring the mighty mushroom along with potatoes and paprika, is partly inspired by the hearty soups of Slovenia, Croatia, Bosnia, Montenegro, and Albania. Both pureed potatoes and yogurt create the creamy texture. Serve with crusty bread on a blustery day to create some cozy comfort and mind relaxation in your kitchen.

In a large Dutch oven or stockpot, heat the olive oil over medium heat. Add the celery and onion and cook, stirring occasionally, until slightly softened, 8 to 10 minutes. Add the mushrooms, sweet paprika, smoked paprika, salt, and black pepper and cook, stirring occasionally, for 5 minutes to give the spices time to flavor the mushrooms. Add the potato and flour and stir for 1 minute, until the flour is coating all the vegetables. Stir in the broth, scraping the sides and bottom to incorporate into the roux mixture. Simmer until the soup just starts to boil, then stir and reduce the heat to medium-low. Add the bay leaf, cover, and simmer, stirring occasionally, for at least 15 minutes, until the potatoes are cooked through (the longer it simmers, the more flavorful and thicker the soup will become).

Turn off the heat. Remove the bay leaf. Slowly whisk in ½ cup yogurt and then the vinegar. Serve in soup bowls dolloped with the remaining yogurt and sprinkled with dill or parsley.

PER SERVING: Calories: 188; Total Fat: 8g; Saturated Fat: 2g; Cholesterol: 6mg; Sodium: 191mg; Total Carbohydrates: 23g; Fiber: 3g; Protein: 9g

Healthy Kitchen Hack: Dried mushrooms are a terrific substitute for some or all of the fresh mushrooms in this soup. They keep for up to a year in your pantry and add incredible concentrated flavor to soups, stews, and sauces. More common dried varieties include shiitake, morel, or porcini. Swap in 3 ounces dried mushrooms for every ½ pound fresh mushrooms. To rehydrate, cover the dried mushrooms with warm water in a bowl and soak for 30 minutes. Rinse the mushrooms to remove any grit. Then soak them in a little bit of olive oil for another 30 minutes to make them silky and less tough before using in your recipe.

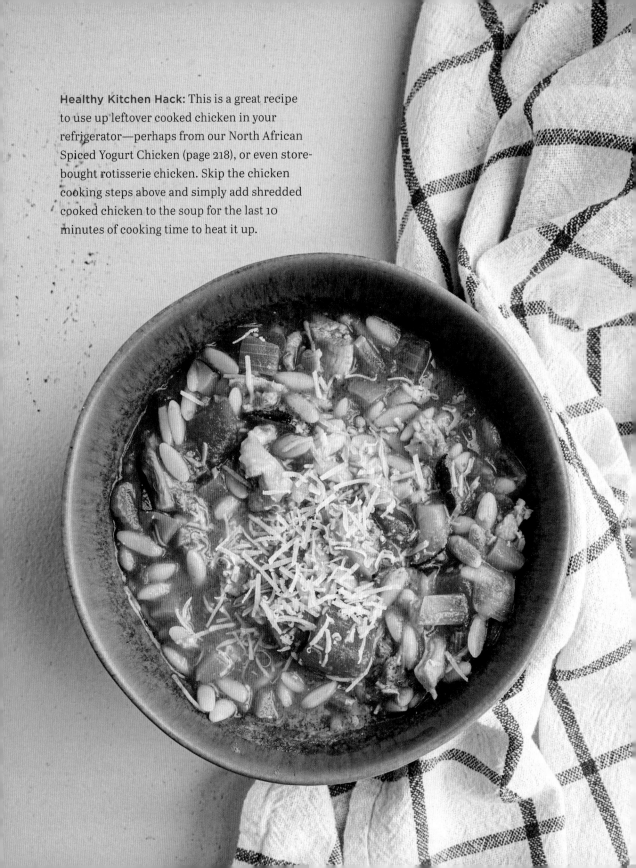

Healthy Kitchen Hack: This is a great recipe to use up leftover cooked chicken in your refrigerator—perhaps from our North African Spiced Yogurt Chicken (page 218), or even store-bought rotisserie chicken. Skip the chicken cooking steps above and simply add shredded cooked chicken to the soup for the last 10 minutes of cooking time to heat it up.

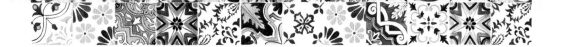

Spicy Turmeric
CHICKEN MINESTRONE SOUP

SERVES 6   Prep time: 15 minutes   ✳   Cook time: 45 minutes

The classic Italian pasta and veggie soup gets a vibrant upgrade in this recipe, with a mix of turmeric and cayenne pepper, two antioxidant-rich spices said to benefit overall brain health. Make it vegetarian by swapping out the chicken for two cans of chickpeas or cannellini beans. This super-filling soup is even better the following day!

- 2 tablespoons extra-virgin olive oil, divided
- 1 pound boneless, skinless chicken breasts, cut into bite-size pieces
- 1 teaspoon ground turmeric, divided
- 1 medium onion, chopped
- 2 carrots, scrubbed and chopped
- 2 celery ribs, chopped
- 1 medium zucchini or summer squash, chopped
- ¼ teaspoon cayenne pepper
- 2 garlic cloves, minced
- 1 (28-ounce) can low-sodium diced tomatoes, undrained
- 6 cups low-sodium chicken or vegetable broth
- ½ (1-pound) package acini de pepe, orzo, or other small pasta shape
- ¼ teaspoon kosher or sea salt
- ¼ teaspoon black pepper
- 3 tablespoons grated Parmesan cheese

Heat 1 tablespoon oil in a large stockpot or Dutch oven over medium heat. Sprinkle the chicken pieces with ½ teaspoon turmeric and add to the pot. Cook, stirring frequently, until the chicken is cooked through and no longer pink in the middle, 8 to 10 minutes. Using a slotted spoon, transfer the chicken to a bowl and set aside.

Heat the remaining 1 tablespoon oil in the pot. Add the onion, carrots, celery, zucchini, remaining ½ teaspoon turmeric, and cayenne pepper and cook, stirring frequently, for 5 minutes. Add the garlic and cook, stirring frequently, for 30 seconds. Stir in the tomatoes with their juices, and cook, stirring occasionally, until the vegetables have softened, about 5 minutes. Add the broth and 1 cup water and turn the heat to medium-high until the liquid starts to boil. Add the pasta, reduce the heat to medium, and cook according to the time on the pasta package. Stir frequently to prevent the pasta from sticking to the bottom.

Return the cooked chicken to the pot, along with the salt and pepper. Stir and cook for at least another 10 minutes, until everything is heated through. Ladle into bowls, sprinkle Parmesan cheese on top, and serve.

PER SERVING: Calories: 392; Total Fat: 10g; Saturated Fat: 2g; Cholesterol: 56mg; Sodium: 386mg; Total Carbohydrates: 46g; Fiber: 5g; Protein: 31g

Tunisian
PEANUT-LENTIL SOUP

SERVES 6 Prep time: 10 minutes ✳ Cook time: 40 minutes

1 cup brown lentils, rinsed

½ onion, chopped

3 garlic cloves,
lightly smashed, divided

1 (2-inch) piece
ginger, peeled and
coarsely chopped
(about 2 tablespoons)

2 teaspoons
smoked paprika

2 teaspoons ground cumin

1 teaspoon caraway seeds

¼ teaspoon kosher
or sea salt

½ cup creamy
peanut butter

2 (14.5-ounce) cans
low-sodium diced
tomatoes, undrained

The warm flavors of cumin, caraway, red chiles, and garlic make up the spicy North African chile paste known as harissa. Inspired by these bold seasonings, this unique, velvety vegan soup features smoked paprika, which contains the hot-tasting capsaicin present in all chiles. Emerging research ties the antioxidant capsaicin with anti-inflammatory properties and potentially lowering the risk for developing Alzheimer's. And garlic is good for memory, so spoon away!

In a large saucepan, combine the lentils, onion, and 2 smashed garlic cloves. Add 3½ cups water and bring to a boil over high heat. Turn the heat to medium-low, cover, and simmer until the lentils are tender, 20 to 25 minutes.

While the lentils cook, combine the remaining smashed garlic clove, ginger, smoked paprika, cumin, caraway seeds, salt, and ⅓ cup water in a blender and puree until smooth. Add the peanut butter and puree until smooth. Pour the pureed mixture into the saucepan with the lentils and add the diced tomatoes with their juices and ½ cup water (to get more flavor from the canned tomatoes, use the water to rinse out the can before you pour it into the pot). Puree the mixture with an immersion blender or carefully transfer it in batches to the stand blender. Heat the pureed soup over medium-low heat until simmering, then cook for 10 minutes for the flavors to blend, stirring occasionally. Serve right away.

PER SERVING: Calories: 310, Total Fat: 12g; Saturated Fat: 2g; Cholesterol: 0mg; Sodium: 396mg; Total Carbohydrates: 42g; Fiber: 8g; Protein: 18g

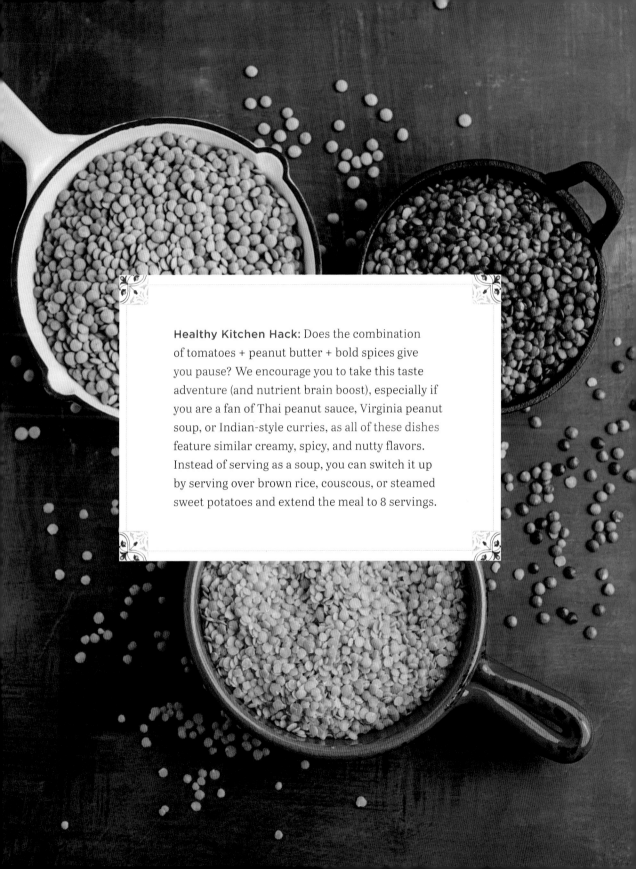

Healthy Kitchen Hack: Does the combination of tomatoes + peanut butter + bold spices give you pause? We encourage you to take this taste adventure (and nutrient brain boost), especially if you are a fan of Thai peanut sauce, Virginia peanut soup, or Indian-style curries, as all of these dishes feature similar creamy, spicy, and nutty flavors. Instead of serving as a soup, you can switch it up by serving over brown rice, couscous, or steamed sweet potatoes and extend the meal to 8 servings.

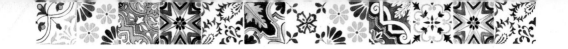

GINGER BUTTERNUT SQUASH SOUP *with Tahini and Toasted Seeds*

SERVES 6 Prep time: 15 minutes ✳ Cook time: 25 minutes

1 tablespoon + 1 teaspoon extra-virgin olive oil, divided

1 medium onion, chopped

2 garlic cloves, minced

1 teaspoon ground ginger, divided

1 teaspoon smoked paprika, divided

½ teaspoon kosher or sea salt, divided

½ teaspoon black pepper, divided

1 (2½- to 3-pound) butternut squash, peeled and cubed, seeds reserved (see Hack)

4 cups low-sodium vegetable broth

½ cup tahini

1 teaspoon rice or white wine vinegar

¼ cup plain 2% Greek yogurt or Homemade Yogurt (page 60)

This Middle Eastern twist on a classic autumn soup will warm you up on those crisp fall days by way of both temperature and spices. Ginger and smoked paprika give gorgeous color, enticing aromas, and a few dashes of antioxidants. Nutty tahini (sesame seed butter) delivers an extra creamy, smooth texture along with the phytonutrient sesamol, which has promising ties to reducing brain plaque and boosting memory. We top this soup off with cool, tangy yogurt paired with homemade toasted and spiced squash seeds (see Hack for substitution ideas).

Preheat the oven to 375°F. Coat a large rimmed baking sheet with cooking spray.

Heat 1 tablespoon oil in a large stockpot over medium heat. Add the onion and cook, stirring occasionally, until just starting to soften, for 5 minutes. Add the garlic, ¾ teaspoon ginger, ¾ teaspoon smoked paprika, ¼ teaspoon salt, and ¼ teaspoon pepper and cook, stirring frequently, for 1 minute. Add the butternut squash and broth and bring to a boil. Turn the heat to medium-low and cook, stirring occasionally, until the squash has softened, about 25 minutes. Turn off the heat.

While the soup cooks, in a medium bowl, mix the remaining ¼ teaspoon ginger, ¼ teaspoon smoked paprika, ¼ teaspoon salt, and ¼ teaspoon pepper. Add the remaining 1 teaspoon oil and the butternut squash seeds and toss well to coat. Spread the seeds evenly on the prepared baking sheet. Bake for 8 minutes, then check the seeds; if they are not yet completely golden brown, continue to bake for an additional 2 to 3 minutes (keep a close eye on the seeds as they burn easily). Cool for 10 minutes.

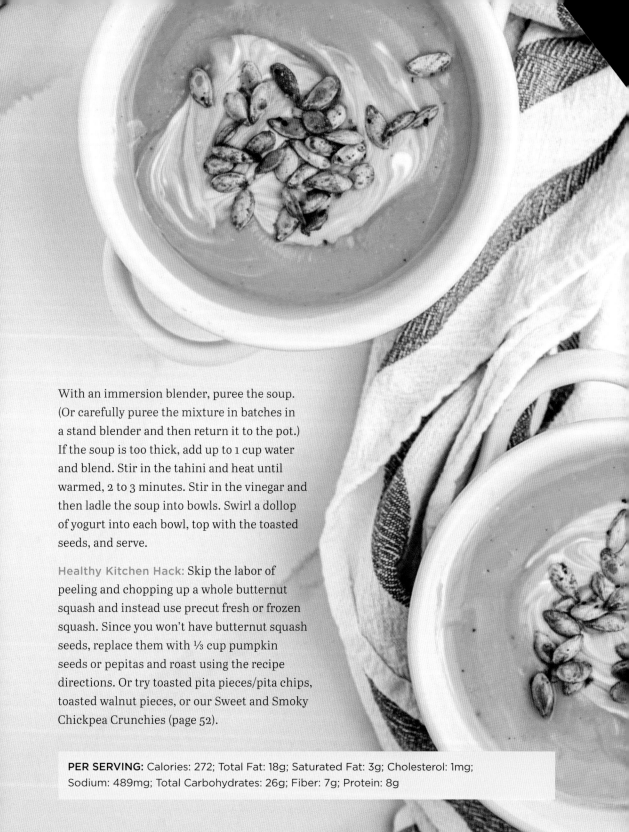

With an immersion blender, puree the soup. (Or carefully puree the mixture in batches in a stand blender and then return it to the pot.) If the soup is too thick, add up to 1 cup water and blend. Stir in the tahini and heat until warmed, 2 to 3 minutes. Stir in the vinegar and then ladle the soup into bowls. Swirl a dollop of yogurt into each bowl, top with the toasted seeds, and serve.

Healthy Kitchen Hack: Skip the labor of peeling and chopping up a whole butternut squash and instead use precut fresh or frozen squash. Since you won't have butternut squash seeds, replace them with ⅓ cup pumpkin seeds or pepitas and roast using the recipe directions. Or try toasted pita pieces/pita chips, toasted walnut pieces, or our Sweet and Smoky Chickpea Crunchies (page 52).

PER SERVING: Calories: 272; Total Fat: 18g; Saturated Fat: 3g; Cholesterol: 1mg; Sodium: 489mg; Total Carbohydrates: 26g; Fiber: 7g; Protein: 8g

STRACCIATELLA SOUP
with Chicken and Spinach

SERVES 4   Prep time: 5 minutes   ❄   Cook time: 15 minutes

4 cups low-sodium chicken broth

1 (10-ounce) package frozen chopped spinach

2 teaspoons dried oregano

¼ teaspoon black pepper, preferably freshly ground

3 large eggs

¼ cup grated Parmesan cheese

1 (12-ounce) can chicken, drained, rinsed, and flaked with a fork, or 1½ cups shredded cooked chicken

1 lemon (optional)

When you swirl an egg into warm broth, kitchen magic occurs as the egg turns into craggy noodle-like formations. Many versions of egg drop soup are stirred up worldwide, and stracciatella is the Italian version. And this recipe showcases how brain foods can be convenience foods: quick-cooking eggs, frozen spinach, and dried herbs make it possible for this pantry-ingredient soup to be ready in a snap.

Pour the broth into a large saucepan or Dutch oven. Add the frozen spinach, oregano, and pepper and bring to a simmer over medium heat, stirring occasionally, until the spinach is thawed, about 10 minutes. Turn the heat down to medium-low.

In a small bowl, whisk together the eggs and cheese. Slowly, in a thin stream, add the egg mixture to the hot soup, stirring gently, until the eggs are set into feathery threads, about 1 minute. Stir in the chicken and cook until heated through, about 2 minutes.

If desired, using a Microplane or citrus zester, grate the zest from the lemon into the soup, then cut the lemon in half and squeeze in 1 tablespoon juice (save the remaining lemon for another use). Serve immediately.

Healthy Kitchen Hack: Frozen spinach is one of our favorite brain foods, packed with the antioxidants lutein and zeaxanthin, which is linked to improved cognitive function in young adults. Add an entire bag or box of it to a pot of almost any canned soup to bump up the nutrition. Or thaw it in the microwave, press out some of the water, and add it to baked pasta recipes, the top of pizza, scrambled eggs, quesadillas, grilled cheese sandwiches, the top of baked potatoes, rice bowls, or bean dishes.

PER SERVING: Calories: 180; Total Fat: 8g; Saturated Fat: 3g; Cholesterol: 183mg; Sodium: 503mg; Total Carbohydrates: 6g; Fiber: 2g; Protein: 21g

TURKISH WHITE BEAN SOUP
with Aleppo Pepper

SERVES 4   Prep time: 5 minutes   ✳ Cook time: 10 minutes

Serena makes this soup when she needs a family-friendly dinner on the table in minutes. She created it to highlight the fruity, tangy, just slightly spicy Aleppo pepper grown in Syria and Turkey—and also after reading about the simple, satisfying white bean and tomato soups of this region. And if you were to custom-design a soup to cut the risk of cognitive decline, this might be it, as its ingredients are all but confirmed to be doing just that, one pleasing spoonful at a time.

In a Dutch oven or large stockpot, heat the oil over medium-low heat. Add the garlic and pepper and cook, stirring occasionally, for 2 minutes, until very fragrant. Add the tomato paste and cook, stirring occasionally, for 3 to 4 minutes, until the paste is nearly incorporated into the oil. Add the beans, salt, and 2½ cups water and stir. Cook until warmed through, 3 to 4 minutes. Stir in the vinegar and top with more pepper. Serve as is, or blend with an immersion blender in the pot or in batches in a stand blender.

Healthy Kitchen Hack: Serena often serves this soup over a pot of pasta to extend it. You could also serve it over a pot of rice or over thick pieces of toasted bread in the bottom of each bowl. And, if you have leftovers, poach an egg in it like shakshuka later in the week.

3 tablespoons extra-virgin olive oil

5 garlic cloves, minced

½ teaspoon Aleppo pepper, plus more for garnish

3 tablespoons tomato paste

2 (15-ounce) cans cannellini beans, drained and rinsed

¼ teaspoon kosher or sea salt

1 tablespoon white wine vinegar or other vinegar

PER SERVING: Calories: 300; Total Fat: 11g; Saturated Fat: 1g; Cholesterol: 0mg; Sodium: 313mg; Total Carbohydrates: 37g; Fiber: 11g; Protein: 13g

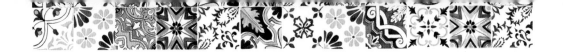

CREAM OF ARTICHOKE SOUP
with Goat Cheese Pita Toasts

SERVES 4   Prep time: 10 minutes   ✹   Cook time: 25 minutes

1 tablespoon extra-virgin olive oil

1 medium onion, chopped

2 garlic cloves, minced

2 (14-ounce) cans artichoke hearts, drained (liquid reserved; see Hack)

1 tablespoon fresh thyme leaves, plus more for garnish

¼ teaspoon kosher or sea salt

¼ teaspoon black pepper

1½ cups low-sodium vegetable broth

1 cup whole milk

2 ounces spreadable goat cheese

1 large pita bread

1 lemon

¼ cup plain 2% Greek yogurt or Homemade Yogurt (page 60)

Simple yet full-bodied, this soup is an easy way to enjoy artichokes—there's no complicated prep as required with fresh artichokes. Egypt, Italy, Spain, and Algeria are among the world's top artichoke producers, and this veggie is featured in even more Mediterranean countries' cuisines. Rich in fiber, folate, and vitamin C, artichokes also provide a healthy dose of vitamin K, which may help protect against aging-related dementia and other cognitive diseases. We top this speedy soup with toasted goat cheese pita pieces for a tangy, creamy bite in every spoonful.

Heat the oil in a large stockpot or Dutch oven over medium heat. Add the onion and cook, stirring frequently, until slightly softened, about 5 minutes. Add the garlic, artichokes, thyme, salt, and pepper and cook, stirring frequently, for 1 minute. Pour in the vegetable broth and ½ cup reserved artichoke liquid. Bring to a boil, then lower the heat to medium-low. Cover and simmer for 10 minutes.

While the soup is simmering, preheat the broiler.

Remove the soup from the heat. Using an immersion blender or a stand blender (blend in two batches), puree until smooth. Return the soup to medium-low heat and whisk in the milk. Reheat for about 5 minutes.

While the blended soup heats, spread the goat cheese on the pita and cut into 4 triangles (to ensure crispy edges). Place the triangles on a rimmed baking sheet and broil until the bread is toasted, watching closely to prevent the bread from burning, 1½ to 2 minutes. Cool slightly, then cut or tear the triangles into ½ inch-pieces.

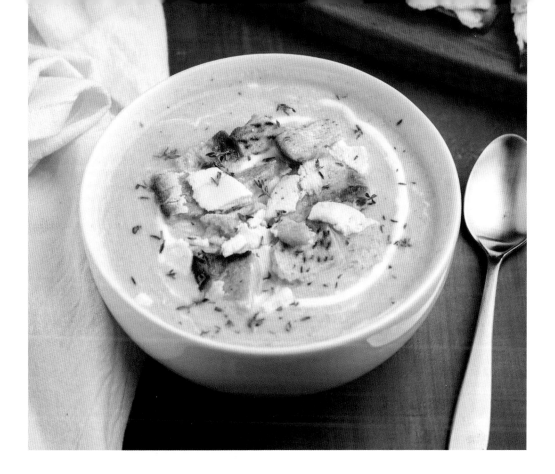

Right before serving, cut the lemon in half and squeeze the juice from one half into the soup. Cut the other half into wedges and set aside. Stir the soup and then ladle it into four bowls. Dollop or swirl with yogurt and sprinkle with extra thyme. Top each bowl with the goat cheese pita toasts and serve with the reserved lemon wedges for squeezing.

Healthy Kitchen Hack: Deanna prefers artichokes that are canned in water, but you can use marinated jarred artichokes here instead. Drain and thoroughly rinse the artichokes, but save the brine for another use (like instant pickled vegetables!). Frozen artichokes work well in this recipe, too. Add about 10 additional minutes to the cooking time so they have time to completely thaw.

PER SERVING: Calories: 227; Total Fat: 10g; Saturated Fat: 4g; Cholesterol: 15mg; Sodium: 559mg; Total Carbohydrates: 25g; Fiber: 5g; Protein: 10g

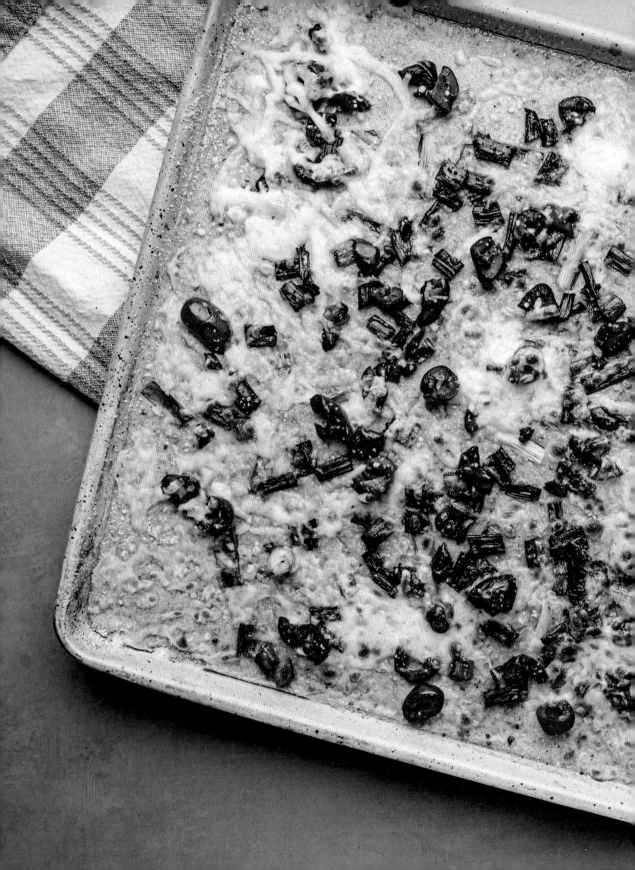

SANDWICHES & PIZZAS

Roasted Veggie and Beet Hummus
SANDWICHES

SERVES 4   Prep time: 20 minutes ✳ Cook time: 15 minutes

3 tablespoons extra-virgin olive oil, divided

1 (15-ounce) can chickpeas, drained (liquid reserved) and rinsed

1 small beet, scrubbed and roughly chopped

2 tablespoons tahini or peanut butter

1 garlic clove, peeled

2 tablespoons pomegranate molasses (see Hack on page 177) or lemon juice

¼ teaspoon kosher or sea salt

1 medium zucchini

8 slices whole-wheat or white bread, toasted if desired

4 large pieces of roasted red peppers (from a 12-ounce jar), drained

If you aren't a fan of cooked beets, we encourage you to try them raw as they are sweeter and less earthy-tasting. (Serena's kids prefer them this way!) Not to mention, raw beets can turn a can of chickpeas into a gorgeous, deep pink hummus in seconds. Plus, this beet and bean combo might even contribute to your cognitive and mental well-being thanks to the 10 grams of fiber per sandwich. Fiber helps keep the gut healthy, and the brain and gut are connected into a seamless system to keep each functioning optimally.

Pour 1 tablespoon olive oil onto a large rimmed baking sheet and place in the oven. Preheat the oven to 400°F with the sheet inside.

Pour the chickpeas into a blender or food processor. Add ¼ cup of the reserved chickpea liquid and process until smooth. Add the beet, remaining 2 tablespoons oil, tahini, garlic, pomegranate molasses, and salt and process until smooth. For a lighter, fluffier texture, add another 1 to 2 tablespoons chickpea liquid to achieve your preferred consistency.

Cut the zucchini in half crosswise, then cut each half lengthwise into ¼-inch-thick planks. Carefully remove the baking sheet from the oven and, using tongs, place the zucchini planks in the hot oil and flip to coat both sides. Roast for 8 to 10 minutes, until just tender. Remove the sheet but keep the oven on.

PER SERVING: Calories: 446; Total Fat: 18g; Saturated Fat: 3g; Cholesterol: 0mg; Sodium: 615mg; Total Carbohydrates: 58g; Fiber: 10g; Protein: 15g

To assemble the sandwiches, spread each slice of bread with 1 tablespoon beet hummus. Layer 4 of the hummus bread slices with 1 slice of zucchini, 1 piece of red pepper, then another slice of zucchini. Top with the remaining beet hummus bread slices. Place the sandwiches on the sheet pan and roast for 2 to 3 minutes, until heated through.

Healthy Kitchen Hack: You can make a rainbow of homemade hummus flavors by following the simple hummus recipe above. Instead of raw beets, add roasted red peppers (red); raw carrots, cooked sweet potato, or canned pumpkin (orange); turmeric (yellow); or thawed frozen peas or fresh cilantro (green).

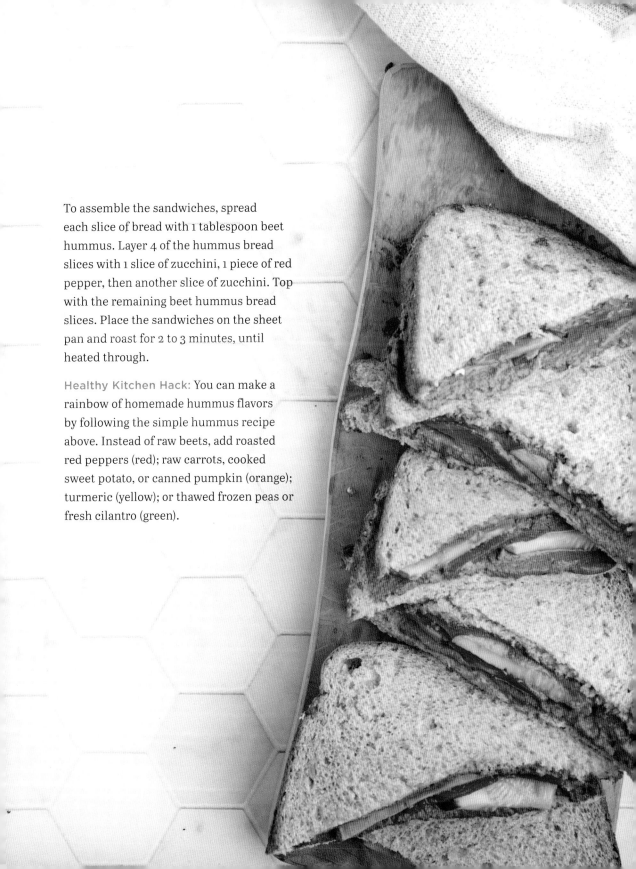

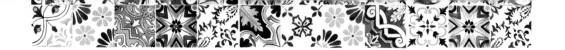

CRISPY EGGPLANT PITAS
with Mediterranean Mayo

SERVES 4   Prep time: 15 minutes   ✳ Cook time: 30 minutes

1 cup panko bread crumbs

1 tablespoon za'atar
(see Hack)

1 large egg

½ teaspoon kosher
or sea salt, divided

1 (1-pound) globe
eggplant, unpeeled and
sliced into ½-inch rounds

1 lemon

½ cup plain
whole-milk Greek yogurt
or Homemade Yogurt
(page 60)

1 tablespoon extra-virgin
olive oil

10–12 fresh mint leaves,
torn

2 whole-wheat pita breads,
halved and toasted

1 cup torn lettuce
or fresh herbs

Years ago, Serena learned that the best way to select an eggplant is to look for one that's "as smooth as a baby's bottom." Having had five babies, she knows a thing or two about that! Her youngest, Zoe, loves eggplant, but the other four...not so much. However, everyone ate up these pita pockets because the crunchy, breaded eggplant is slathered in our Mediterranean mayo made up of creamy, luxurious olive oil and mint-infused yogurt. And now that you know the selection trick, you can shop smartly for eggplant, which is full of anthocyanins, the brain-enhancing antioxidants with a purple color.

Preheat the oven to 425°F. Spread a sheet of parchment paper on a large rimmed baking sheet.

In a wide, shallow bowl, use a fork to mix the panko and za'atar. (Note: Make sure your za'atar contains salt; if not, add ⅛ teaspoon to the panko mixture.) In a shallow bowl, whisk together the egg, ¼ teaspoon salt, and 1 tablespoon water.

Dredge each eggplant round in the egg mixture, then place in the bread crumbs and cover, pressing gently to stick and then shaking off any excess. Place the breaded rounds on the prepared baking sheet. Bake for 20 minutes. Flip all the slices and continue to bake until golden and crispy, an additional 10 to 12 minutes.

Meanwhile, using a Microplane or citrus zester, grate the zest from the lemon into a medium bowl, then cut the lemon in half and squeeze in 1 tablespoon juice (save the remaining lemon for another use). Whisk in the yogurt, oil, mint, and remaining ¼ teaspoon salt.

Fill each pita bread half with the eggplant slices, the mayo, and lettuce and serve immediately.

Healthy Kitchen Hack: Don't have za'atar in your spice drawer? Make your own mix! In a small dry skillet, toast 3 tablespoons sesame seeds over medium-low heat, stirring occasionally, until fragrant, about 2 minutes. Pour the seeds into a mini food processor and add 2 tablespoons dried oregano, 2 tablespoons dried thyme, and ½ teaspoon kosher or sea salt. Using a Microplane or citrus zester, grate the zest from 1 lemon into the food processor. Pulse a few times to combine, then pour into a jar. When completely cool, screw on the lid. Store at room temperature and use within a month.

> *The minty mayo made our pita sandwiches great. My husband liked it better than regular mayo. I will be making that mayo all the time now!*
>
> AMY FROM
> ST. LOUIS, MO

PER SERVING: Calories: 271; Total Fat: 8g; Saturated Fat: 2g; Cholesterol: 51mg; Sodium: 438mg; Total Carbohydrates: 42g; Fiber: 7g; Protein: 11g

Chef Lorenzo's
SNACK SANDWICHES

SERVES 6   Prep time: 10 minutes   ✻   Cook time: 5 minutes

2 tablespoons extra-virgin olive oil, divided

2 teaspoons lemon juice

¼ teaspoon black pepper

⅛ teaspoon kosher or sea salt

1 (5-ounce) package arugula or baby lettuce (about 2 cups)

1 (12-ounce) loaf ciabatta or Italian bread, halved lengthwise

1 garlic clove, cut in half

3 ounces prosciutto or very thinly sliced deli ham

A few years ago during a cooking demo, Serena was lucky enough to work with Chef Lorenzo, who grew up in Bologna. He made her his favorite after-school snack, which inspired this simple yet succulent sandwich recipe. Meal or snack time, we think you'll love our version of his childhood memory, which also features two of our favorite brain-benefiting ingredients: garlic and olive oil.

Place the top oven rack about 4 inches below the broiler element. Preheat the broiler.

In a medium bowl, whisk together 1 tablespoon oil, the lemon juice, pepper, and salt. Add the arugula and toss. Set aside.

Arrange the bread halves cut side up on a large rimmed baking sheet. Broil for 1 to 2 minutes, until the bread just begins to turn golden brown, turning halfway through (watch carefully to avoid burning).

Rub a garlic half firmly on the cut sides of each toasted bread slice (save the garlic halves for another use). Brush with the remaining 1 tablespoon olive oil.

Arrange the prosciutto on the toasted sides of both bread halves. Top one half with the arugula mixture. Quickly flip the other prosciutto-layered bread half onto the arugula.

To serve, slice the sandwich into six even sections.

Healthy Kitchen Hack: Skip the mayo or other sandwich spreads and instead use this mix of greens, lemon juice, olive oil, salt, and black pepper for any sandwich, from tuna to cheese to egg salad. The tart, salty tangle of lettuces is so flavorful, you may find yourself using a double portion of fiber and antioxidant-rich greens between the bread slices.

PER SERVING: Calories: 203, Total Fat: 7g; Saturated Fat: 1g; Cholesterol: 8mg; Sodium: 602mg; Total Carbohydrates: 28g; Fiber: 1g; Protein: 9g

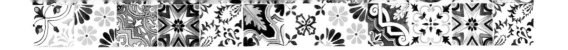

PROVENÇAL GRILLED CHEESE
with Walnut Mustard Spread

SERVES 4   Prep time: 10 minutes   ❊   Cook time: 20 minutes

Here's a thought that's good for mental health: sitting down at a lovely French café to an extra crispy, melty grilled cheese. As you make this sandwich in your "café" kitchen, you'll pile on ingredients that can be good for your brain health as well as your taste buds. Walnuts, olive oil, and mustard seeds all have potential benefits. Like all seeds, mustard seeds are rich in every component needed to become a whole plant, and their bold flavor signals the presence of strong polyphenols (plant antioxidants). Shop for whole-grain Dijon mustard for more seed power!

1 lemon

½ cup coarsely chopped walnuts (about 2 ounces)

1 garlic clove, peeled

2 tablespoons extra-virgin olive oil, divided

1 tablespoon whole-grain Dijon mustard

1 teaspoon herbes de Provence, plus more for garnish (see Hack)

8 thin slices crusty white sourdough bread, toasted

4 ounces Brie cheese, cut into 8 thin slices

1 large tomato, sliced and seeded

Using a Microplane or citrus zester, grate the zest from the lemon into a blender or mini food processor, then cut the lemon in half and squeeze in 1 tablespoon juice (save the remaining lemon for another use). Add the walnuts, garlic, 1 tablespoon oil, the mustard, and 3 tablespoons water and puree until thick and creamy. Add the herbes de Provence and pulse to combine. (Add another 1 to 2 tablespoons water to thin out the spread, if desired.)

Heat a cast-iron or other large, heavy skillet over medium heat for 5 to 10 minutes, until very hot.

Brush one side of all the toast slices with the remaining 1 tablespoon oil, then flip them over. Spread the other side of each slice with 1 teaspoon of the walnut mustard (reserve the remaining spread). On the mustard side, layer four of the toasts with a cheese slice, a tomato slice, and then another cheese slice. Top with the remaining toast slices, mustard side down and oil side up.

continued on page 119

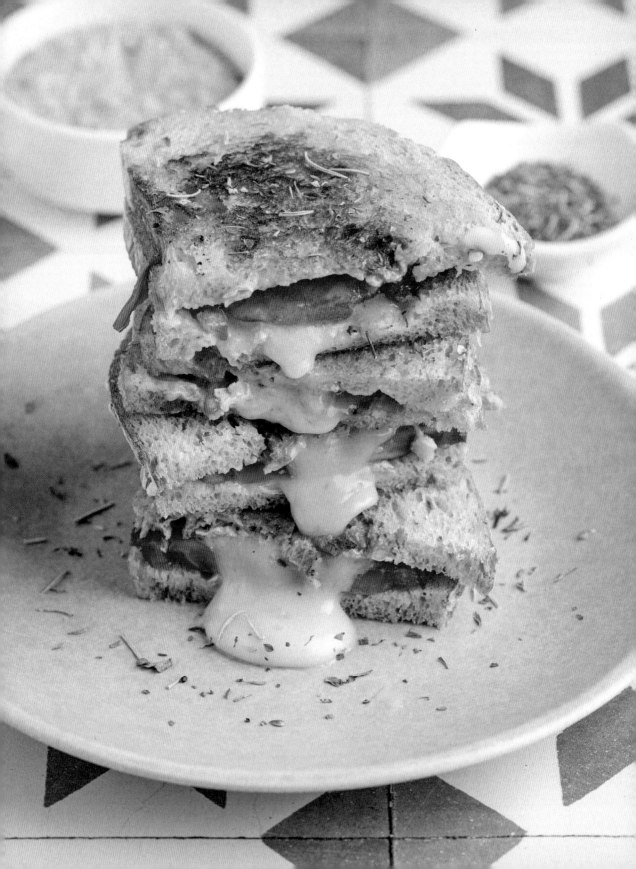

continued from page 117

Add two sandwiches to the hot skillet and cook for 3 minutes, until golden brown. Flip with a spatula and cook for an additional 2 to 3 minutes. Repeat with the other two sandwiches. Sprinkle with additional herbs de Provence and serve immediately with the remaining mustard on the side.

Tip: To prevent a soggy sandwich, pat dry the tomato slices after removing the seeds and use no more than 1 teaspoon of mustard per toast slice.

Healthy Kitchen Hack: Herbes de Provence is the iconic dried herb mixture used in many traditional Southern France dishes. You can buy it premade or make it yourself! Combine 1 tablespoon of each of the following dried herbs: thyme, oregano, basil, rosemary, and tarragon (or fennel seed). Sprinkle on grilled meats and fish, fold into scrambled eggs, mix into bean and lentil dishes, whip into ricotta cheese, blend into vinaigrettes, and sprinkle on salads.

PER SERVING: Calories: 362; Total Fat: 25g; Saturated Fat: 7g; Cholesterol: 28mg; Sodium: 568mg; Total Carbohydrates: 26g; Fiber: 2g; Protein: 12g

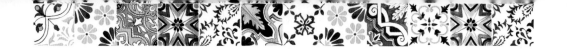

Smarter PIZZA DOUGH

SERVES 8 Prep time: 20 minutes

3 cups all-purpose flour, plus more for kneading

1 tablespoon baking powder

¾ teaspoon kosher or sea salt

1 cup plain 2% Greek yogurt or Homemade Yogurt (page 60)

3 tablespoons extra-virgin olive oil

Over the years of recipe testing for cookbooks, we feel like we've finally perfected our speedy pizza dough. Yogurt and baking powder stands in for leavening of yeast, while the olive oil yields a smoother and more stretchable dough. Featured in our Caprese Salad Pizza (page 122) and Three-Cheese Pizza with Sweet Potato (page 124), this recipe can also be used to make flatbread (see Hack).

In a large bowl or stand mixer bowl, combine the flour, baking powder, and salt. With a wooden spoon or spatula if mixing by hand or the dough hook attachment if using a stand mixer, mix the dry ingredients. Add the yogurt, ⅓ cup at a time, stirring after each addition. Add the olive oil and 3 tablespoons water and continue to mix until a slightly shaggy dough begins to form. If the dough is too dry and does not come together, add 1 or 2 additional tablespoons of water.

Knead the dough on a lightly flour-dusted work surface for 2 to 3 minutes, until smooth (if the dough is too sticky, add a few teaspoons of flour to the surface and work it in). Form the dough into a ball, cover with a dish towel, and let rest for at least 10 minutes before using. For baking directions, see the recipes for Caprese Salad Pizza (page 122) and Three-Cheese Pizza with Sweet Potato (page 124), or use it to make flatbreads (see Hack).

Tip: The recipe makes about 1½ pounds of dough and can be used to make two large pizzas or eight individual pizzas. If not using right away, store the dough after resting in an airtight container in the freezer for up to 6 months. Defrost by letting the dough sit on the counter for a few hours until completely thawed.

66

I was skeptical if this no-rise dough would work and taste good, but it really did! It was so easy to make, too.

LARRY FROM TYLER, TX

PER SERVING: Calories: 237; Total Fat: 6g; Saturated Fat: 1g; Cholesterol: 3mg; Sodium: 192mg; Total Carbohydrates: 38g; Fiber: 1g; Protein: 8g

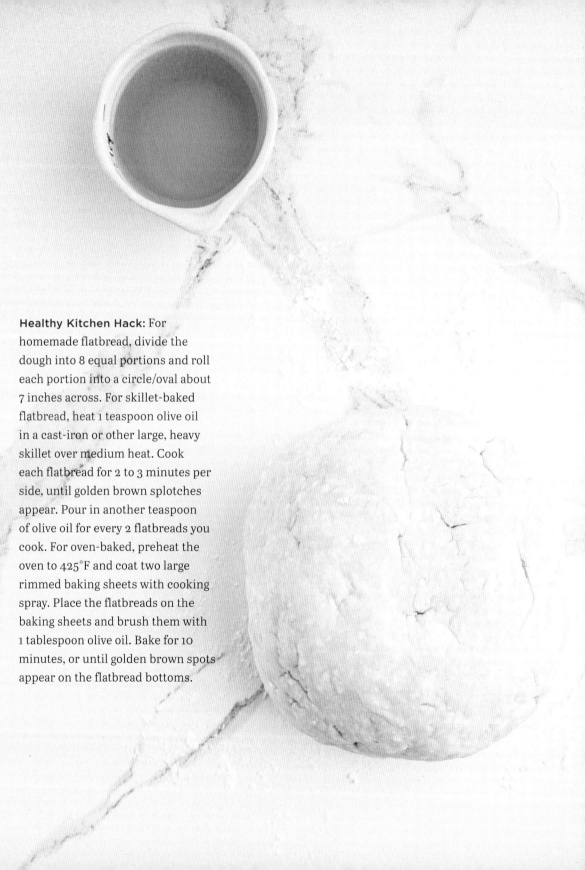

Healthy Kitchen Hack: For homemade flatbread, divide the dough into 8 equal portions and roll each portion into a circle/oval about 7 inches across. For skillet-baked flatbread, heat 1 teaspoon olive oil in a cast-iron or other large, heavy skillet over medium heat. Cook each flatbread for 2 to 3 minutes per side, until golden brown splotches appear. Pour in another teaspoon of olive oil for every 2 flatbreads you cook. For oven-baked, preheat the oven to 425°F and coat two large rimmed baking sheets with cooking spray. Place the flatbreads on the baking sheets and brush them with 1 tablespoon olive oil. Bake for 10 minutes, or until golden brown spots appear on the flatbread bottoms.

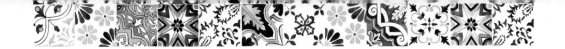

Caprese SALAD PIZZA

SERVES 8 (makes two 13-inch pizzas) — Prep time: 15 minutes ✳ Cook time: 20 minutes

1 recipe Smarter Pizza
Dough (page 120) or
1 to 1½ pounds
store-bought pizza dough
(see Hack), at room
temperature

2 tablespoons extra-virgin
olive oil, divided

1 tablespoon
balsamic vinegar or
pomegranate molasses
(see Hack on page 177)

¼ teaspoon kosher
or sea salt

1 pint cherry tomatoes,
halved

8 ounces fresh
mozzarella cheese,
thinly sliced and torn
into 1-inch pieces

2 cups arugula
or baby spinach

½ cup fresh basil leaves,
torn

1 tablespoon capers,
drained

We love Caprese salad—the classic combo of ripe tomatoes, fresh mozzarella, and basil—so much that we "spread" it over dough to make this salad pizza. The result is a topping of sweet blistered tomatoes, melted mozzarella, and a pile of greens with tangy capers dressed in tart balsamic vinaigrette. Arugula's bold flavor is a signal that it contains a good amount of antioxidants. Researchers even think that the activation of bitter taste receptors may have beneficial effects on the brain.

Arrange the oven racks in the upper-middle and lower-middle positions. Preheat the oven to 475°F. Line two large rimmed baking sheets with parchment paper. Lightly flour your work surface, and divide the dough into two equal portions. Roll each portion into a circle/oval 12 or 13 inches across (it doesn't have to be perfectly round) and place on the lined baking sheets. Brush the pizza crusts with ½ tablespoon oil. Set aside.

In a large bowl, whisk together the remaining 1½ tablespoons oil, vinegar, and salt.

Put the tomatoes in another bowl and drizzle with about half of the oil and vinegar mixture, then toss to coat. Scatter the tomatoes and mozzarella cheese over both pizzas.

Bake for 15 to 18 minutes, until the edges of the crust start to turn golden brown.

To the bowl with the remaining vinegar and oil, add the arugula, basil, and capers and toss to coat. Scatter this salad over both pizzas, including the dressing in the bottom of the bowl.

Cut each pizza into 8 slices and serve immediately.

PER SERVING: Calories: 348; Total Fat: 15g; Saturated Fat: 5g; Cholesterol: 18mg; Sodium: 363mg; Total Carbohydrates: 40g; Fiber: 2g; Protein: 13g

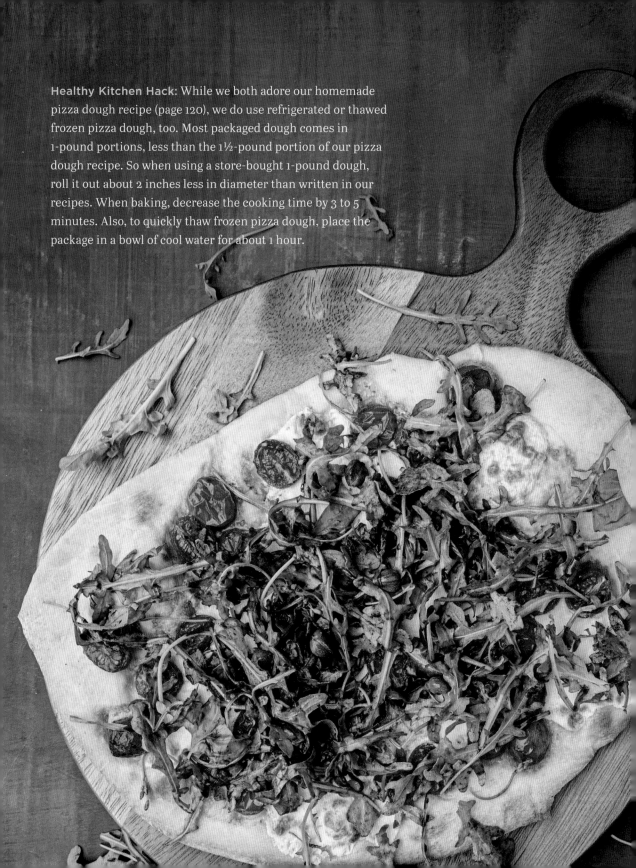

Healthy Kitchen Hack: While we both adore our homemade pizza dough recipe (page 120), we do use refrigerated or thawed frozen pizza dough, too. Most packaged dough comes in 1-pound portions, less than the 1½-pound portion of our pizza dough recipe. So when using a store-bought 1-pound dough, roll it out about 2 inches less in diameter than written in our recipes. When baking, decrease the cooking time by 3 to 5 minutes. Also, to quickly thaw frozen pizza dough, place the package in a bowl of cool water for about 1 hour.

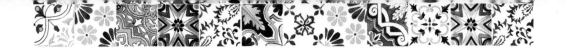

THREE-CHEESE PIZZA
with Sweet Potato

SERVES 8 (makes two 13-inch pizzas) Prep time: 15 minutes ✳ Cook time: 30 minutes

3 tablespoons extra-virgin olive oil, divided

3 tablespoons chopped fresh chives, divided

1 tablespoon chopped fresh rosemary

¼ teaspoon kosher or sea salt

¼ teaspoon black pepper

1 small sweet potato, scrubbed, halved lengthwise, and sliced crosswise into ¼-inch-thick half circles

1 pound mushrooms (such as button, cremini, and/or others), sliced

1 recipe Smarter Pizza Dough (page 120) or 1 to 1½ pounds premade pizza dough, at room temperature (see Hack on page 123)

8 ounces whole-milk ricotta

⅛–¼ teaspoon crushed red pepper (optional)

3 ounces provolone cheese, sliced or shredded

¼ cup grated Parmesan or Pecorino Romano cheese

Bursting with vital nutrients, including fiber, potassium, and vitamins A and C, the humble sweet potato turns out to be a worthy pizza topping. Its starchy sweetness is a lovely balance to earthy mushrooms and fresh herbs. And not surprisingly (because we're featuring it in this book!), those sweet potato nutrients can help lower inflammation and improve memory as we age.

Arrange the oven racks in the upper-middle and lower-middle positions. Preheat the oven to 475°F.

In a large bowl, combine 1 tablespoon oil, 2 tablespoons chives, the rosemary, salt, and black pepper. Add the sweet potato slices and toss to coat. Arrange the slices on a large rimmed baking sheet (there will be some herbs left in the bowl). Add another 1 tablespoon oil to the bowl, then toss in the mushrooms. Spread them out onto another large rimmed baking sheet. Roast the sweet potatoes and mushrooms for 10 to 12 minutes, until the sweet potato slices are mostly softened. Remove both sheets from the oven.

While the vegetables cook, lightly flour your work surface, and divide the dough into two equal portions. Roll each portion into a circle/oval 12 to 13 inches across (it doesn't have to be perfectly round) and place on separate sheets of parchment paper. Brush each pizza crust with the remaining 1 tablespoon oil and set aside.

In a small bowl, whisk together the ricotta, remaining 1 tablespoon chives, and crushed red pepper, if using.

Remove the sweet potato slices and mushrooms from the baking sheets and transfer to two medium bowls. With a dish towel, carefully wipe clean any moisture from the sheets, then place the parchment with the pizza crusts on the separate sheets. Arrange the provolone cheese over both pizza crusts. Scatter with the mushrooms. Dollop the chive ricotta onto each pizza, then top with the sliced sweet potatoes. Sprinkle with the Parmesan cheese.

Bake for 17 to 20 minutes, until the edges of the crust start to turn golden brown. Cut each pizza into 8 slices and serve immediately.

Healthy Kitchen Hack: Tap into your freezer and pantry if you don't have fresh sweet potatoes or mushrooms on hand. Frozen sweet potato fries make a convenient swap for fresh pizza toppings. Heat in the microwave on a microwave-safe plate, covered with a moist paper towel, for about 2 minutes. Or heat up in an air fryer at 400°F for 5 minutes; shake the basket and then cook for another 5 minutes. Canned mushrooms, drained and patted dry, can also sub in for their fresh counterparts.

> 66
> *I wasn't sure about this combination of toppings, but it came out really well—especially the yummy pairing of provolone, ricotta, and Parmesan.*
>
> KENDAHL FROM MINNEAPOLIS, MN

PER SERVING: Calories: 409; Total Fat: 19g; Saturated Fat: 7g; Cholesterol: 27mg; Sodium: 436mg; Total Carbohydrates: 44g; Fiber: 3g; Protein: 15g

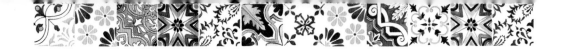

SCALLION FLATBREAD
with Mozzarella and Olives

SERVES 4 Prep time: 15 minutes ✳ Cook time: 15 minutes

2 tablespoons
yellow cornmeal

1 bunch (8–9) scallions
(green onions), green
and white parts

¾ cup all-purpose flour

¾ cup whole-wheat flour

1 tablespoon
dried oregano

½ teaspoon baking powder

½ teaspoon kosher
or sea salt

1 cup plus 2 tablespoons
2% milk

2 large eggs

2 tablespoons extra-virgin
olive oil

½ cup chopped
black olives (such as
Kalamata, Niçoise,
and/or canned black)

1½ cups shredded
part-skim mozzarella
cheese

¼ teaspoon black pepper

This is how Serena's mom makes flatbreads—with an easy "pour pizza" dough that has baked-in flavor. Bright green scallions are sprinkled into the dough before baking and sautéed into a rich oil that's drizzled on top with more fresh scallions. And the brain benefits are abundant from the fiber in the whole-wheat flour and scallions, memory-boosting choline in the eggs, and good fats from the olives and olive oil.

Place the top oven rack about 4 inches below the broiler element. Preheat the oven to 400°F. Coat a large rimmed baking sheet well with cooking spray. Sprinkle the sheet with cornmeal, then turn and tap the baking sheet to spread the cornmeal evenly over the surface.

Slice half of the scallions into 1-inch pieces. On a separate section of the cutting board, thinly slice the remaining scallions into ¼-inch pieces. Set aside.

In a large bowl, whisk together the flours, oregano, baking powder, and salt. In a small bowl, whisk together the milk and eggs. Add the milk mixture to the flour mixture and whisk until well combined.

Pour the batter onto the prepared baking sheet and spread it into an even layer (it's fine if some of the cornmeal gets mixed into the batter). Sprinkle with the 1-inch scallion pieces.

Bake on any oven rack for 10 to 12 minutes, until the crust appears dry in the center. Remove from the oven and turn on the broiler.

While the flatbread cooks, heat the oil in a large skillet over medium heat. Add the ¼-inch scallion pieces to the hot oil (reserving about 2 tablespoons on the cutting board for

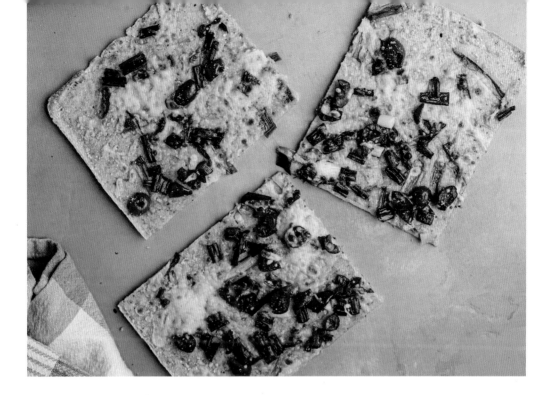

final topping). Cook, stirring occasionally, for 5 minutes, until about half of them get crispy with brown edges. Evenly spread the cooked scallions and all the oil in the pan over the baked crust. Sprinkle with the olives, then with the cheese.

Place the flatbread on the upper oven rack under the broiler. Broil, rotating the pan halfway through (and watching carefully to prevent burning), for 2 to 3 minutes total, until the cheese is toasted.

Sprinkle with black pepper and garnish with the reserved fresh scallions. Serve warm or at room temperature, sliced into 4 or 8 pieces.

Healthy Kitchen Hack: We love scallions, or green onions as they're also called. When we have two or three leftover from a bunch, we like to slice them and use them up in the following ways:

> Stir into jarred salsa to freshen it up.

> Mix with sliced cucumber, a spoonful of vinegar, and a shake of salt and sugar, to make a quick cuke salad.

> Sprinkle over soups or into sandwich fillings.

66

The whole-wheat crust of the flatbread was our favorite part. Also, this was a very easy and quick recipe to make.

EVIE FROM
BILLINGS, MT

PER SERVING: Calories: 434; Total Fat: 20g; Saturated Fat: 7g; Cholesterol: 120mg; Sodium: 690mg; Total Carbohydrates: 47g; Fiber: 5g; Protein: 19g

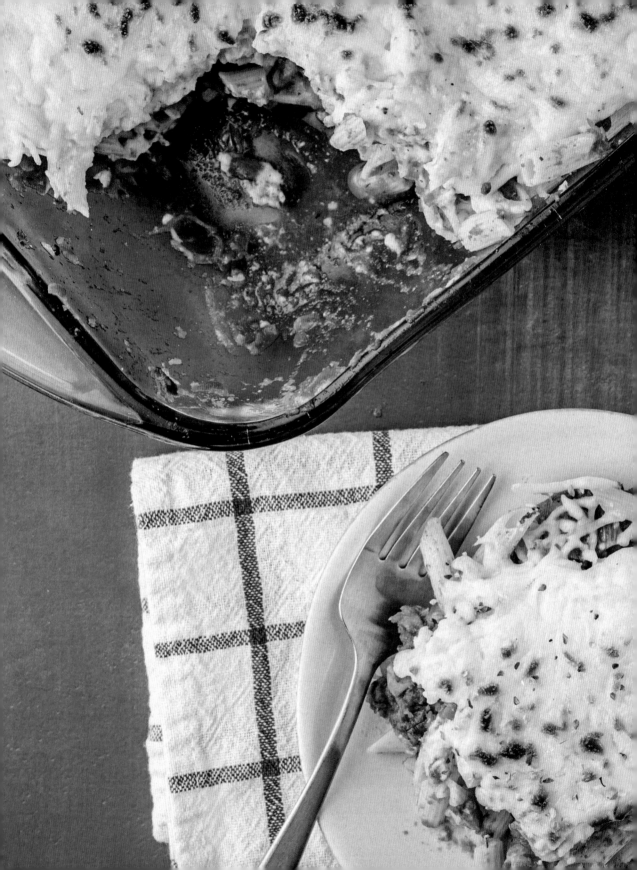

PASTA

Speedy PESTO SAUCE

SERVES 8 (makes about ¾ cup) Prep time: 10 minutes

2 cups fresh greens
or herb leaves and stems
(such as arugula, spinach,
basil, mint, parsley,
or cilantro)

¼ cup nuts or seeds
(such as walnuts,
pecans, almonds,
pistachios, peanuts,
and/or sunflower seeds)

3 tablespoons grated
aged cheese (such as
Parmesan, Pecorino
Romano, Asiago,
or cheddar)

2 garlic cloves, peeled

¼ teaspoon kosher
or sea salt

¼ cup extra-virgin olive oil

No time to cook up pasta sauce? No problem! With this pesto "formula," you can mix and match your favorite ingredients or do what we do: blend together whatever delicate greens, nuts, and aged cheese you have on hand at the moment. Pesto is classically served with pasta, but it also makes an excellent sandwich spread, pizza sauce, flavor bomb for vegetable soup, or aromatic topping for fish like our Quick Fish with Walnut-Arugula Pesto (page 180).

Combine the greens, nuts, cheese, garlic, and salt in a blender or food processor. Process until the pesto is roughly chopped. Scrape down the sides of the blender. Replace the blender lid but remove the middle of the lid. Turn the blender back on and slowly drizzle in the olive oil; process until smooth.

Use right away or store in an airtight container in the refrigerator for up to 1 week.

Healthy Kitchen Hack: One of the best tools in your brain-healthy kitchen? Your freezer! Though we use nuts often because of their strong ties to brain health, we store them in the freezer to keep them fresher longer. Freezing your pesto will make it last even longer than storing it in the fridge. Spoon 1-tablespoon portions into each compartment of an ice cube tray and freeze. Once frozen, transfer the cubes to a freezer bag or airtight container. To defrost, simply add frozen pesto cubes to hot pasta or soup and mix. To defrost as a spread, microwave in 10-second increments until thawed.

PER SERVING: (1½ tablespoons): Calories: 96; Total Fat: 10g; Saturated Fat: 2g; Cholesterol: 1mg; Sodium: 77mg; Total Carbohydrates: 1g; Fiber: 1g; Protein: 2g (Note: Nutritional values will vary based on greens, nuts/seeds, and cheese used.)

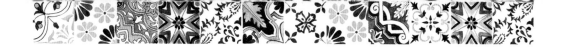

Pasta CECI E BROCCOLINI

SERVES 4 Prep time: 10 minutes ❋ Cook time: 20 minutes

For generations, Italian families have been making endless variations of this simple bean-and-pasta-based comfort food dish, which is one of the many mouthwatering vegan pasta recipes you can find in sunny Mediterranean places where dairy is sometimes less common. Our version of pasta ceci (Italian for chickpeas) builds big flavor with smooth garlic oil, crispy garlic chips, a bit of red pepper, robust broccolini, and tart lemon. Chickpeas and other legumes are good sources of vitamin B6, niacin, and folate, and getting all the B-complex vitamins may ease stress and boost mood. This is Serena's very favorite dish in this book, so it certainly improves her mood!

1 lemon

1¾ teaspoons kosher or sea salt, divided

½ (1-pound) package rotini or other medium-size pasta (such as orecchiette, fusilli, penne, or cavatappi)

2 tablespoons extra-virgin olive oil

5 garlic cloves, sliced

8 ounces broccolini or broccoli, stems and florets cut into long, slim pieces, patted dry

¼ teaspoon crushed red pepper

1 (15-ounce) can chickpeas, drained (liquid reserved) and rinsed

¼ teaspoon black pepper

Using a Microplane or citrus zester, grate the zest from the lemon into a small bowl, then cut the lemon in half and squeeze in the juice from one half. Cut the other half into wedges for serving and set aside.

Fill a large stockpot with water. Cover and bring to a boil over high heat. Add 1½ teaspoons salt and then stir in the pasta. Cook, stirring occasionally, for 1 to 2 minutes short of al dente according to the package instructions.

While the pasta cooks, pour the oil into a large skillet or a Dutch oven. Add the garlic slices to the oil in a single layer. Turn the heat to medium and cook, stirring occasionally, until a few garlic chips are crisp and golden brown, about 5 minutes. (Avoid overcooking.) Using a slotted spoon, transfer the garlic to a plate. Place the skillet with the oil back over medium heat and add the broccolini and red pepper. Cook undisturbed until a few broccolini turn golden, then stir occasionally until tender-crisp, about 5 minutes total. Add the chickpeas and cook for 1 minute to warm through. Turn off the heat until the pasta is ready.

continued on page 133

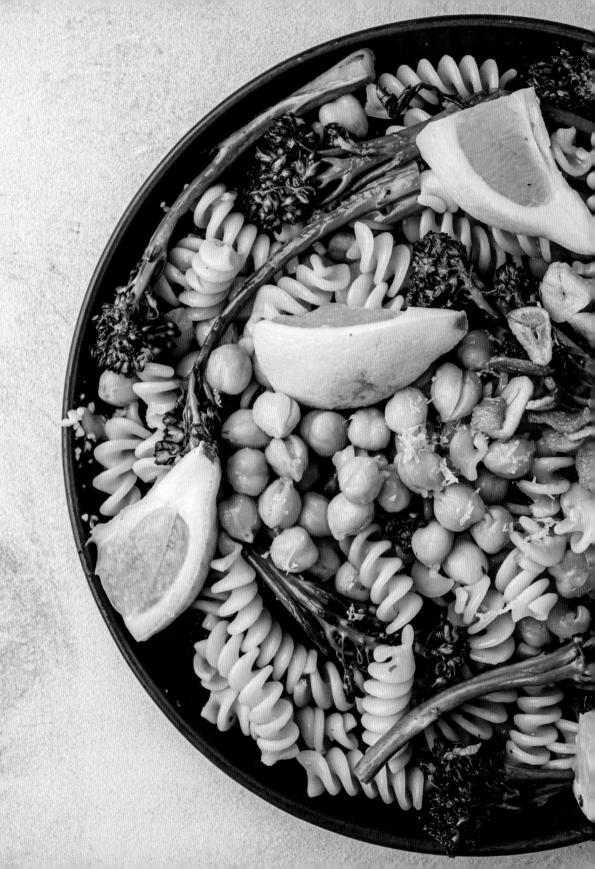

continued from page 131

Use a slotted spoon or kitchen spider to transfer the cooked pasta to the skillet; reserve the pasta cooking water in the pot.

Turn the heat to medium and add the remaining ¼ teaspoon salt, ½ cup reserved chickpea liquid, and ¼ cup pasta water. Cook, stirring, until only a little liquid remains (about 2 tablespoons), 2 to 3 minutes. Add the lemon juice with zest and the black pepper and toss to combine. Remove from the heat, top with the garlic chips, and serve warm with the lemon wedges for squeezing.

Healthy Kitchen Hack: While we love cheese with all our hearts, we know that some folks can't or don't eat it. So to add the salty, umami flavors of aged cheese, roast up some garlic instead. Start with a whole head of garlic and remove most of the papery skins on the outside. Slice ¼ inch off the top of the head and wrap the head in aluminum foil. Roast in a 400°F oven for about 50 minutes, until the garlic cloves are soft and spreadable. Once cool enough to handle, squeeze the cloves out of the skins onto a small plate. Sprinkle with ⅛ teaspoon kosher or sea salt, mash with a fork, and stir into 1 to 2 tablespoons olive oil. Drizzle into any dish you typically would sprinkle with cheese.

PER SERVING: Calories: 397; Total Fat: 10g; Saturated Fat: 1g; Cholesterol: 0mg; Sodium: 389mg; Total Carbohydrates: 63g; Fiber: 8g; Protein: 15g

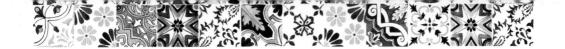

Smart and Spicy
SUMMER SPAGHETTI

SERVES 4   Prep time: 10 minutes   ✳ Cook time: 15 minutes

1½ teaspoons kosher
or sea salt

½ (1-pound) package
spaghetti

2 tablespoons extra-virgin
olive oil

1 small onion, diced

2 garlic cloves, minced

½ teaspoon crushed
red pepper, plus more
for serving (optional)

1 large tomato, chopped,
or 1 (14.5-ounce) can
low-sodium diced
tomatoes, undrained

6 tablespoons grated
Parmesan cheese, divided

¼ cup fresh basil leaves,
torn

We make a version of this spaghetti all'arrabbiata (Italian for "angry" sauce) all summer long when fresh tomatoes are having their moment in the sun. Consider it more of a template to add whatever is on hand or may be fresh from the garden, like onions, bell peppers, zucchini, green beans, peas, and more. The hefty kick of heat comes from red pepper flakes, but other spicy Mediterranean seasonings like harissa, Aleppo pepper, or smoked paprika can easily be swapped in. Chiles get their heat from capsaicin, the mighty anti-inflammatory antioxidant tied to decreased risk for cognitive decline. It may also reduce stress and depression by triggering the release of feel-good endorphins. So, perhaps we should rename it spaghetti "buon umore" (good mood)!

Fill a large stockpot with water. Cover and bring to a boil over high heat. Add the salt and then stir in the pasta. Cook, stirring occasionally, until al dente according to the package instructions.

While the pasta cooks, heat the oil in a large skillet over medium heat. Add the onion and cook, stirring frequently, until it just starts to soften, about 5 minutes. Add the garlic and red pepper flakes and cook, stirring frequently, for 1 minute. Add the tomatoes with their juices and let simmer, stirring occasionally, until the pasta is done, but no more than 5 minutes. (If the sauce starts to boil at any point, reduce the heat to medium-low.)

Transfer ¼ cup pasta water directly from the stockpot to the skillet and stir until everything is mixed well. Using tongs, transfer the cooked spaghetti to the skillet and toss to coat (keep the pasta water in the pot). Stir until the liquid is almost all absorbed, about 1 minute, and then stir in an additional 2 to 4 tablespoons reserved pasta water until the sauce reaches your preferred consistency. Add ¼ cup of the cheese and mix well. Remove from the heat.

Mix in the remaining 2 tablespoons cheese and toss well until the pasta is coated. Top the pasta with the basil and more crushed red pepper, if desired. Serve immediately.

Healthy Kitchen Hack: For another layer of flavor (and maybe some heat!), add roasted sweet bell peppers and/or fresh chiles (like poblano, jalapeño, serrano, etc.). Cut each pepper in half lengthwise and remove the stem, seeds, and white membrane. Place skin side up on a foil-lined baking sheet and press to flatten. Broil until the skins are black and blistered, 5 to 8 minutes (depending on the size of the chiles). Remove from the oven, cover completely with the foil, and let sit for at least 10 minutes or until cool enough to handle. Remove the skins, chop up the pieces, and add to this recipe with the tomatoes. Refrigerate any leftovers in an airtight container.

PER SERVING: Calories: 329; Total Fat: 10g; Saturated Fat: 3g; Cholesterol: 5mg; Sodium: 282mg; Total Carbohydrates: 49g; Fiber: 3g; Protein: 11g

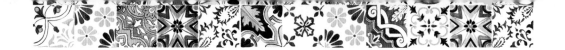

FETTUCCINE
with Prosciutto, Prunes, and Black Pepper

SERVES 4 Prep time: 15 minutes ✳ Cook time: 20 minutes

1½ teaspoons kosher or sea salt

½ (1-pound) package fettuccine

2 tablespoons extra-virgin olive oil

½ red onion, thinly sliced in half rings

2 ounces prosciutto, thinly sliced

8 pitted prunes, chopped

1 teaspoon freshly ground black pepper, plus more for serving (optional)

½ cup grated Parmesan cheese, divided

> 66
> *I really loved the way the different ingredients all came together. I've made it several times since and it may be one of my favorite pasta dishes of all time!*
>
> NICOLE FROM
> TOWN BANK, NJ

Intrigued by a pasta recipe calling for dates, Deanna swapped in the prunes she had in her pantry and—long story short—she created one of her very favorite dishes, ever! While pairing dried fruit with pasta might not seem typical, Mediterranean cuisines regularly match grains with the intense natural sweetness of dried fruit to balance out other flavors—here, salty prosciutto, savory Parmesan, and spicy black pepper. Dried fruit like prunes can enhance a dish's appearance and serve as a concentrated source of vitamins and minerals that help maintain brain health and mental activity.

Fill a large stockpot with water. Cover and bring to a boil over high heat. Add the salt and then stir in the pasta. Cook, stirring occasionally, until al dente according to the package instructions.

While the pasta cooks, heat the oil in a large skillet over medium heat. Add the onion and cook, stirring frequently, until softened, 5 minutes. Add the prosciutto and cook, stirring frequently, until crispy, 3 minutes. Add the prunes and black pepper and cook, stirring frequently, until fragrant, 2 minutes. Add ⅓ cup reserved pasta water and stir until everything is mixed well. Using tongs, transfer the cooked fettuccine to the skillet and toss to coat. Stir frequently until the liquid is almost all absorbed, about 1 minute, and then add an additional ⅓ cup reserved pasta water. Continue to stir frequently until almost all the liquid is absorbed, about another minute. Add ¼ cup cheese and mix well. Mix in 2 to 3 additional tablespoons reserved pasta water to help incorporate the cheese and toss well. Remove from the heat.

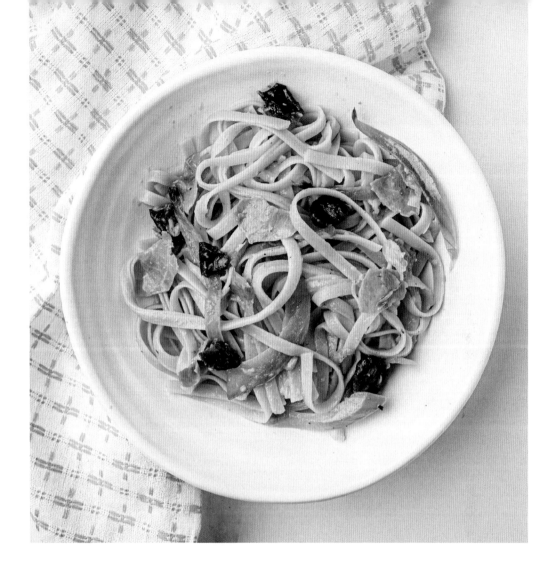

Mix in the remaining ¼ cup cheese; toss well until the pasta
is coated and almost all the liquid is absorbed. Top the pasta
with more black pepper, if desired. Serve immediately.

Healthy Kitchen Hack: Experiment with other chopped
dried fruit in this recipe. Pitted dates, dried figs, or golden
raisins are all fabulous flavor swaps for the prunes. And
if you have different types of peppercorns, like red, pink,
green, or white, try those here, too.

PER SERVING: Calories: 409; Total Fat: 12g; Saturated Fat: 4g; Cholesterol: 10mg;
Sodium: 569mg; Total Carbohydrates: 61g; Fiber: 2g; Protein: 16g

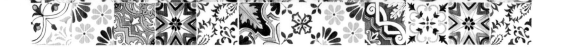

Save-the-Day
SLOW COOKER LASAGNA

SERVES 8   Prep time: 25 minutes   ❋   Cook time: 3 to 6 hours

1 pound lean ground beef and/or lamb

1 medium onion, chopped

3 garlic cloves, minced

1 teaspoon fennel seeds

¼ teaspoon crushed red pepper

¼ teaspoon kosher or sea salt

1 (24-ounce) jar low-sodium tomato sauce

1 (6-ounce) can tomato paste

2 cups shredded part-skim mozzarella cheese, divided

1½ cups whole-milk ricotta or cottage cheese

2 cups finely chopped or shredded mixed vegetables, such as zucchini, broccoli, cauliflower, celery, spinach and/or peas

1 tablespoon dried oregano

½ teaspoon black pepper

9 regular (not "no boil") lasagna noodles

¼ cup grated Parmesan or Pecorino Romano cheese

At the end of a long day of activities, you can "save the day" by immediately sitting down to a big (crock) pot of Mediterranean comfort food for dinner. This type of layered pasta dish with a bit of meat and cheese was originally served in Treviso, Italy. Our version is quicker to assemble than lots of lasagna recipes—also, you won't have to seek out those special no-boil noodles. After many tries, Serena perfected the proportion of liquid to noodles to get them al dente, but not mushy, as can happen in the slow cooker. Beef and lamb contain zinc, and getting enough of that mineral may help clear foggy thinking and memory problems. All these colorful veggies and the tomato sauce are rich in inflammation-fighting beta-carotene.

In a large skillet, cook the ground beef and onion over medium heat, occasionally stirring and breaking up the chunks of meat, until the meat begins to brown, 5 minutes. Add the garlic, fennel seeds, red pepper, and salt and continue to cook, stirring occasionally, until the onion is tender and the meat is browned, about 5 more minutes. Turn the heat up to medium-high and stir in the pasta sauce, tomato paste, and 1 cup water (from rinsing out the empty jar). Bring to a boil and then turn off the heat.

While the meat cooks, in a medium bowl, stir together 1½ cups mozzarella, the ricotta, vegetables, oregano, and black pepper.

To assemble the lasagna, coat a 6- or 7-quart slow cooker with cooking spray. Spoon one-fourth of the meat sauce into the slow cooker. Top with 3 noodles, breaking them to cover most of the surface. Top with one-third of the mozzarella mixture. Repeat the layers two more times, and end with the remaining meat sauce. Sprinkle the remaining ½ cup mozzarella cheese and the Parmesan over the top.

Cover and cook on high for 2½ hours or on low for 5 to 6 hours, then turn off the slow cooker and let the lasagna set for 20 minutes before serving.

Healthy Kitchen Hack: Since this recipe uses half of a box of lasagna noodles, here are some ideas on what to do with the rest of them: Boil the noodles according to the package directions and make lasagna soup: lasagna noodles, ricotta, and diced veggies mixed in tomato soup, then topped with mozzarella. Or break up the noodles, boil, and serve in place of any recipe calling for smaller pasta shapes. Or simply save them to make lasagna again another day!

66

I really like the convenience of slow cooker lasagna! And this one is so substantial with so many layers and lots of veggies, I didn't even need to make a side salad.

CHERYL FROM PITTSFIELD, MA

PER SERVING: Calories: 436; Total Fat: 18g; Saturated Fat: 9g; Cholesterol: 76mg; Sodium: 584 mg; Total Carbohydrates: 39g; Fiber: 4g; Protein: 29g

MARINATED EGGPLANT FUSILLI
with Feta and Mint

SERVES 8 Prep time: 30 minutes ✳ Cook time: 20 minutes

4 ounces feta or fresh mozzarella cheese in brine

1 (1-pound) globe eggplant, unpeeled and cut into ¾-inch cubes

1½ teaspoons kosher or sea salt

1 (1-pound) package fusilli or other medium pasta (such as orecchiette, penne, rotini, or cavatappi)

2 tablespoons extra-virgin olive oil

4 garlic cloves, minced

½ teaspoon black pepper

1 large tomato, chopped, or 1 (14.5-ounce) can low-sodium diced tomatoes, drained (liquid saved for another use)

⅓ cup fresh mint leaves, torn

When you bring this corkscrew pasta dish to the table, it's up to you if you want to share the secret ingredient. Young cheeses like feta and fresh mozzarella are packaged in liquid that's a gold mine of flavor, yet usually it's just dumped. But using that brine infuses your dish with the salty creaminess of the cheese—in this recipe, it adds flavor to your sauce and takes the eggplant from bland to bold. Eggplant is a good source of potassium, which helps keep your brain's electrical signals and communication system working properly throughout your life. Beyond marinating brain-boosting veggies for extra flavor, feta and mozzarella brine can have many uses; see the Hack for ideas.

Drain the liquid from the feta into a small bowl and reserve it. Crumble the feta and set aside in a separate small bowl.

Put the eggplant in a shallow bowl. Drizzle with 2 tablespoons feta brine and toss to combine well. Let sit for 15 minutes. Drain the eggplant (discard the brine) and pat dry with a clean towel.

Meanwhile, fill a large stockpot with water. Cover and bring to a boil over high heat. Add the salt and then stir in the pasta. Cook, stirring occasionally, until 1 minute short of al dente according to the package instructions. Using a kitchen spider or a slotted spoon, transfer the pasta to a bowl; reserve the pasta cooking water in the pot.

PER SERVING: Calories: 303; Total Fat: 8g; Saturated Fat: 3g; Cholesterol: 13mg; Sodium: 445mg; Total Carbohydrates: 49g; Fiber: 4g; Protein: 10g (Note: Sodium value will vary depending on cheese variety.)

Heat the oil in a Dutch oven or large skillet over medium-high heat. Add the eggplant and cook, stirring occasionally, for 5 minutes, until softened. Reduce the heat to medium, add the garlic, and cook, stirring frequently, until fragrant, 1 minute. Add the cooked pasta along with ¼ cup reserved pasta water and 3 tablespoons feta brine and toss to coat. Stir frequently, until the liquid is almost all absorbed, 1 to 2 minutes. Add the pepper and reserved feta and stir to combine. Remove from the heat. Stir in the tomatoes and mint and serve immediately.

Healthy Kitchen Hack: Besides this recipe, use feta or fresh mozzarella brine to add flavor in these ways: Marinate any part of a chicken for 15 to 30 minutes. Mix a few tablespoons of brine into your homemade vinaigrette dressing. Add fresh-cut veggies to the brine and "pickle" them for a few hours or overnight. Stir 2 to 3 tablespoons into our Smarter Pizza Dough on page 120 (and add a little more flour if the dough is sticky). And remember, fresh cheese brines are very salty, so there's no need to add salt to these recipe ideas.

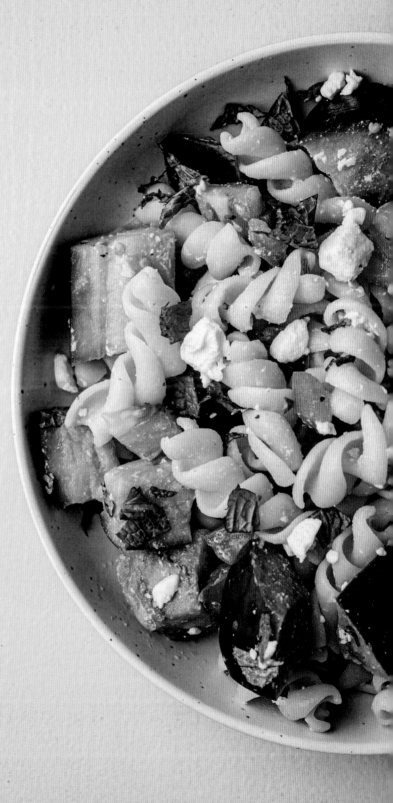

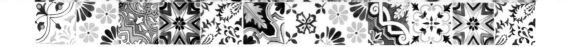

OVEN-BAKED GNOCCHI
with Lemon–Black Pepper Sauce

SERVES 4 Prep time: 15 minutes ✳ Cook time: 30 minutes

1 lemon

1 (2-ounce) can anchovies packed in olive oil, undrained

1 tablespoon extra-virgin olive oil

2 garlic cloves, minced

1 (1-pound) package frozen potato or ricotta gnocchi (not thawed)

1 (14-ounce) can artichokes hearts, drained, rinsed, and chopped

¼ teaspoon black pepper

2 tablespoons grated Parmesan cheese

¼ cup fresh basil leaves, torn

One of Deanna's favorite pasta tricks is to put frozen gnocchi directly into a baking pan and cook them in the oven casserole-style. Ingredient inspiration for this dish came from her recent trip to Provence, where she enjoyed two culinary highlights: anchoïade (the classic Provençal dip made up of anchovies, olive oil, vinegar, and garlic) and artichokes prepared many ways. Since these ingredients are also staples of Italian cuisine—and high on the list of foods with cognitive health ties—pairing them with pasta makes perfect "smart" sense.

Preheat the oven to 450°F.

Using a Microplane or citrus zester, grate the zest from the lemon into a 9 × 13-inch metal baking pan, then cut the lemon in half and squeeze in 1 tablespoon juice (save the remaining lemon for another use). Set aside.

Using a fork, remove 6 anchovies from the tin and set aside (save the remaining anchovies for another use). Pour all the oil from the tin into a small saucepan, add the additional 1 tablespoon olive oil, and heat over medium heat. Add the garlic and cook, stirring constantly, for 30 seconds. Reduce the heat to medium-low and add the anchovies; cook, stirring frequently and mashing them up with the back of a spoon, for 1 minute. Continue to cook, stirring occasionally, for 4 more minutes, until the anchovies "melt" into the oil.

Pour the anchovy-garlic oil into the baking pan (be sure to scrape all the bits from the bottom of the pot into the pan), then whisk with the lemon zest and juice. Add the frozen gnocchi, artichokes, and pepper and gently mix all the ingredients together.

Bake for 12 minutes, stirring halfway through the cooking time. After 12 minutes, carefully add 1 cup water to the pan and stir. Sprinkle with the cheese and bake for another 10 to 12 minutes, until a thick sauce forms. Stir to coat all the gnocchi with the sauce as it will continue to thicken. Sprinkle with the basil and serve warm.

Healthy Kitchen Hack: Get your green on with this gnocchi dish! Add any delicate leafy greens like spinach or arugula, or toss in heartier greens like kale, collards, or Swiss chard with the ribs/stems removed and finely chopped, along with the chopped leaves. Mix in with the gnocchi and artichokes and bake according to the directions. Or mix in the frozen version of those greens (thawed and drained).

PER SERVING: Calories: 344; Total Fat: 9g; Saturated Fat: 2g; Cholesterol: 21mg; Sodium: 659mg; Total Carbohydrates: 54g; Fiber: 3g; Protein: 13g

ROMAN-STYLE GNOCCHI
with Olives and Thyme

SERVES 6   Prep time: 15 minutes   ✳ Cook time: 25 minutes

4 cups 2% milk

⅛ teaspoon kosher or sea salt

1½ cups semolina flour (see Hack)

3 tablespoons unsalted butter

⅔ cup grated Parmesan or Pecorino Romano cheese, divided

2 large egg yolks, lightly beaten

½ (6-ounce) can pitted green or black olives, chopped or sliced (about 25 olives)

2 tablespoons extra-virgin olive oil

2 tablespoons chopped fresh thyme

¼ teaspoon ground black pepper

You won't believe how easy it is to whip up homemade pasta when you make this quintessential Italian comfort food dish! Unlike the more common potato gnocchi, gnocchi alla Romana are made with semolina flour, shaped into wide flat circles, and typically baked (instead of boiled) with cheese and butter. We bake up these gnocchi with a double dose of olives—olive oil and chopped olives—for a rich, buttery flavor with brain-friendly benefits.

In a large saucepan, bring the milk and salt to a simmer over medium heat. Slowly pour in the semolina flour and cook, whisking constantly, for 2 minutes. Reduce the heat to medium-low, switch to a wooden spoon, and stir frequently until a thick dough forms, about another 8 minutes (it will require some arm strength to stir!). Remove from the heat.

Preheat the oven to 425°F. Coat two 9 × 13-inch baking pans or casserole dishes with cooking spray.

Add the butter to the saucepan with the semolina dough and stir until it melts, then mix in ⅓ cup grated cheese. Add one egg yolk at a time, thoroughly mixing until the dough becomes smooth and slightly glossy. Dump the dough onto a large, rimmed baking sheet (or a clean countertop) and, using your hands or the back of a silicone spatula, press and spread the dough in an even layer about ½ inch thick (the dough will fill up just about the entire sheet). Using a 3-inch round cookie cutter, mason jar lid, or mouth of a drinking glass, cut into rounds and arrange in the baking pans (the gnocchi can slightly overlap each other). Take the remaining dough scraps, press them together, and flatten the dough to a ½-inch thickness again. Cut more rounds and repeat the process until all the dough is used up and arranged in

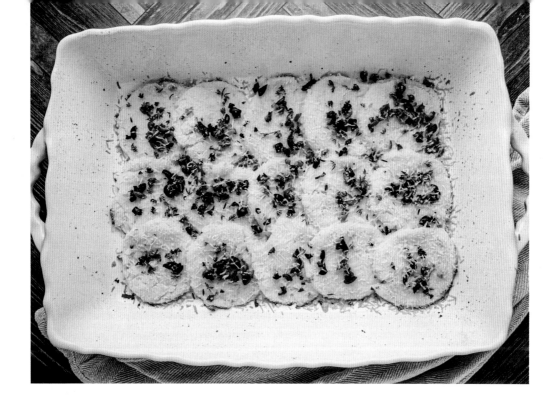

the baking pans (you should end up with 30 to 34 gnocchi). Sprinkle the gnocchi with the olives and remaining ⅓ cup cheese and drizzle with the olive oil.

Bake for 12 to 15 minutes, until the gnocchi start to turn golden brown. Top with the thyme and pepper and serve.

Healthy Kitchen Hack: Semolina flour is made from durum wheat (which is different from common bread wheat) and is popular in Italy for pasta making and in North Africa for making couscous. Since it's milled from the endosperm, the inner part of the wheat kernel, semolina is packed with high-quality, brain-friendly nutrients like B vitamins (especially folate), protein, iron, selenium, fiber, magnesium—the list goes on. Besides serving them with olives, try topping your semolina gnocchi with tomato sauce, our Pan-Roasted Mushrooms in Wine and Thyme (page 86), or our Ratatouille with Socca (page 160).

The instructions on making this type of gnocchi were clear and easy. My entire family loved them!

DAWN FROM
HAVERTOWN, PA

PER SERVING: Calories: 395; Total Fat: 20g; Saturated Fat: 9g; Cholesterol: 96mg; Sodium: 382mg; Total Carbohydrates: 40g; Fiber: 2g; Protein: 15g

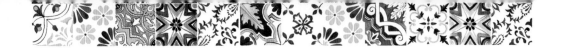

Shortcut
HOMEMADE RAVIOLI

SERVES 6   Prep time: 25 minutes   ✳   Cook time: 25 minutes

2 cups shredded part-skim mozzarella cheese

1 cup whole-milk ricotta

1 teaspoon freshly grated nutmeg or ½ teaspoon ground nutmeg (see Hack)

1 (12-ounce) package wonton wrappers (see Tip)

1 teaspoon kosher or sea salt

2 tablespoons extra-virgin olive oil

2 garlic cloves, lightly smashed

⅓ cup coarsely chopped walnuts

1 teaspoon vinegar (any type)

6 fresh sage leaves, torn

¼ teaspoon black pepper (preferably freshly ground)

Store-bought wonton wrappers make homemade pasta a breeze. Whenever Serena makes these ravioli, her children watch eagerly. As soon as she scoops them from the water, they only get a minute to cool before the kids start popping them, still steaming, into their mouths. When the cooked ravioli aren't coming fast enough, the children help stuff them and it becomes a little kitchen party. Get your own ravioli assembly line going with your loved ones (and if your party participants are older, have the line end with a glass of wine)! This cooking camaraderie is good for mental health—and so are the walnuts and olive oil that top these melty cheese ravioli.

Line two large rimmed baking sheets with parchment paper.

In a medium bowl, stir together the mozzarella, ricotta, and nutmeg.

Fill a small bowl with water and put it near your work surface. Place one wonton wrapper on a dry surface. (Keep the remaining wonton wrappers in the package while you work so they don't dry out.) Spoon 2 teaspoons of the cheese filling into the center of the wonton. Dip your finger in the water and run it along the edges of the wonton wrapper to make the wrapper sticky. Place another wrapper on top, then firmly press the edges together to seal. Place the sealed ravioli on one of the lined baking sheets. Repeat with the remaining wonton wrappers and filling, to make 24 ravioli.

When close to finishing filling the ravioli, fill a large pot or Dutch oven with about 2 inches of water and add the salt. Bring it to a simmer over medium heat. Scoop about ½ cup of the hot water into a large serving platter to warm it and place it near the stove.

Gently slide 6 ravioli into the simmering water in the pot. Stir once very gently to keep the ravioli from sticking to the bottom and to each other, and cook for 3 minutes, until warmed through.

Dump the hot water out of the platter. Using a kitchen spider or slotted spoon, transfer the ravioli to the serving platter. Cook the remaining ravioli, 6 at a time, and add them to the bowl along with a few tablespoons of hot water to keep them warm and prevent sticking.

While the ravioli cook, heat the oil in a large skillet over medium heat. Add the garlic and cook for 1 to 2 minutes, until fragrant and just beginning to turn slightly yellow. Remove the garlic from the oil (and save to use in another recipe, if desired). Add the walnuts to the garlic oil in the skillet and toast for 1 to 2 minutes, until fragrant. Stir in the vinegar and sage leaves. Spoon the flavored oil over the ravioli. Top with the black pepper and serve immediately.

Tip: Wonton wrappers are typically in the refrigerated produce section next to the tofu.

Healthy Kitchen Hack: Fresh nutmeg is preferable for this recipe as its earthy flavor complements the creamy cheese filling and fresh sage. Use a Microplane to grate a whole nutmeg (it looks like a large nut). Freshly grated nutmeg is light and very fluffy, so it takes less to fill a measuring spoon. Heavier ground nutmeg from a spice jar is denser and more potent, which is why we call for only half as much.

66

Yum! The carbs, cheese, nuttiness, and spice are right up my alley, especially for a cozy fall dish.

MEGAN FROM
HIGHLAND, IL

PER SERVING: Calories: 386; Total Fat: 20g; Saturated Fat: 8g; Cholesterol: 40mg; Sodium: 540mg; Total Carbohydrates: 36g; Fiber: 1g; Protein: 18g

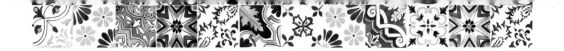

MUSHROOM PASTITSIO
"Baked" Pasta

SERVES 8 Prep time: 40 minutes ❋ Cook time: 25 minutes

- 3 tablespoons extra-virgin olive oil, divided
- 1 pound mushrooms (such as button, cremini, and/or others), finely chopped
- 1 medium onion, chopped
- 1 medium carrot, scrubbed and shredded
- ¼ cup dry red wine or 1 tablespoon red wine vinegar plus 3 tablespoons water
- 1 tablespoon dried oregano
- ½ teaspoon ground cinnamon
- 1 (28-ounce) can low-sodium crushed tomatoes
- 1¾ teaspoons kosher or sea salt, divided
- 1 (1-pound) package penne
- 2 tablespoons white whole-wheat or all-purpose flour
- 2 cups 2% milk, warmed for 1 minute in the microwave
- ¼ teaspoon black pepper
- ¼ teaspoon ground nutmeg (preferably freshly grated)
- 2 large egg yolks
- 2 cups shredded part-skim mozzarella cheese

Often called Greek lasagna, pastitsio is soul-satisfying to eat in the way that hearty baked pasta dishes are. But with our version, we use the broiler to shortcut the finish and toast the signature béchamel cheese sauce topping to a dark golden brown. (We simplified that béchamel, too.) The warm cinnamon-scented tomato sauce is also rich in the brain-friendly nutrient lycopene.

Place the top oven rack about 4 inches below the broiler element. Preheat the oven to 200°F. Coat a 9 × 13-inch broiler-safe baking pan with cooking spray.

Heat 1 tablespoon oil in a Dutch oven or large saucepan over medium-high heat. Add the mushrooms, onion, and carrot and cook, stirring occasionally, until they soften and most of the liquid evaporates, 10 minutes. Add the red wine, oregano, and cinnamon and cook, stirring occasionally, until the liquid evaporates, 2 to 3 minutes. Add the tomatoes and cook, stirring occasionally, until the mixture boils. Turn the heat down to medium and cook for 5 minutes, until slightly thickened. Turn off the heat and cover to keep warm.

Meanwhile, fill a large stockpot with water. Cover and bring to a boil over high heat. Add 1½ teaspoons salt and then stir in the pasta. Cook, stirring occasionally, until 1 to 2 minutes short of al dente according to the package instructions. Drain the pasta and transfer to the prepared baking pan. Return the empty pot to the stove.

Pour the tomato sauce over the pasta and stir to combine. Place in the oven to keep warm.

To make the white sauce, heat the remaining 2 tablespoons oil in the same pot over medium heat. Sprinkle the flour

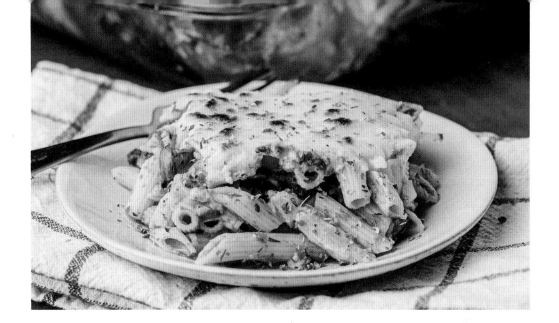

over the oil and whisk until well combined, about 1 minute. Slowly pour in the warm milk while whisking constantly, keep whisking as you bring it just to a boil; the sauce will begin to thicken. Remove from the heat and whisk in the remaining ¼ teaspoon salt, the pepper, and nutmeg.

In a medium bowl, whisk the egg yolks, then whisk in about 1 cup of the white sauce until incorporated. Add the warm egg mixture to the pot and bring to a boil, stirring constantly. Boil, still stirring, for 1 minute, or until the sauce thickens and can coat the back of a spoon.

Remove the pasta from the oven and turn on the broiler. Pour the white sauce in an even layer over the pasta and sprinkle with the cheese. Broil, rotating the pan halfway through (and watching carefully to prevent burning), for 1 to 2 minutes total, until the topping turns a speckled, dark golden brown—almost burnt looking. Remove from the oven and let sit for 10 minutes before serving.

Healthy Kitchen Hack: Got kids who don't love mushrooms? Get them involved in mushroom prep as they might be more willing to try them. Have kids help wash mushrooms by "floating them down the river" like mini boats (yes, you should wash your mushrooms!). Let them use a wire egg slicer to slice mushrooms.

> 66
> *We are familiar with traditional pastitsio. And my family really liked this version! My husband even ate it for breakfast and lunch the next day.*
>
> HILARY FROM LANCASTER, PA

PER SERVING: Calories: 445; Total Fat: 13g; Saturated Fat: 5g; Cholesterol: 65mg; Sodium: 407mg; Total Carbohydrates: 62g; Fiber: 5g; Protein: 21g

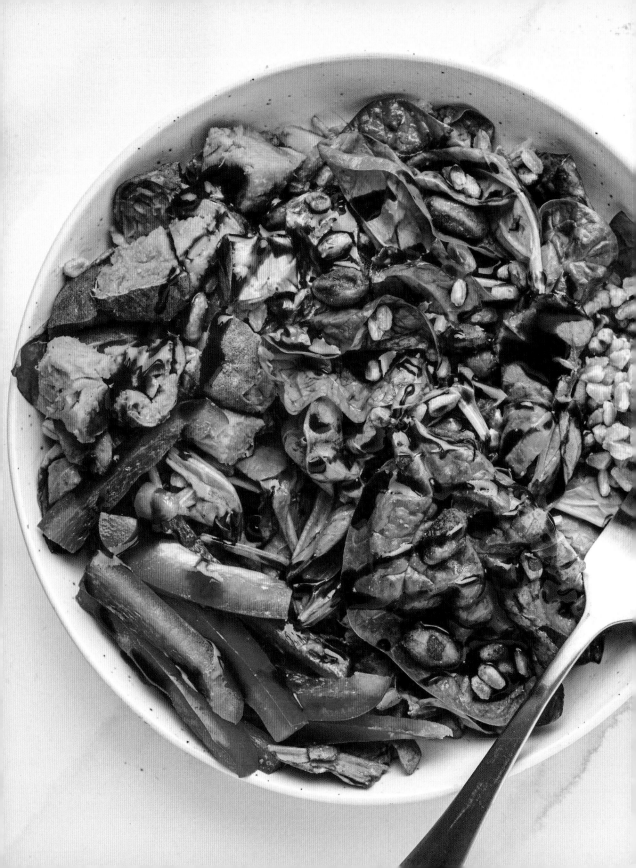

VEGETARIAN MAIN DISHES

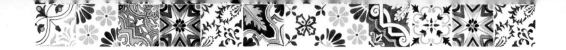

SPEEDY PAELLA
with Cauliflower Rice

SERVES 4 Prep time: 10 minutes ✳ Cook time: 25 minutes

2 tablespoons extra-virgin olive oil, divided

1 tablespoon balsamic vinegar

1 tablespoon Dijon mustard

½ teaspoon smoked paprika

½ teaspoon kosher or sea salt, divided

¼ teaspoon black pepper

1 small head cauliflower (about 1 pound), cut into ½-inch florets

1 large bell pepper (any color), seeded and chopped

4 garlic cloves, minced

1 teaspoon ground turmeric

2 cups instant brown rice

2 cups low-sodium vegetable broth

1 (14.5-ounce) can low-sodium diced tomatoes, undrained

1 cup frozen peas

½ cup pitted green olives, halved, 2 tablespoons liquid reserved

1 lemon, cut into wedges

Here's our speedy vegan riff on paella, the beloved Spanish rice dish from the Valencia region. We roast cauliflower with seasonings found in the spicy Spanish sausage chorizo and swap in instant brown rice for the longer cooking, short-grain Bomba rice. And while saffron traditionally flavors paella, it's expensive, so instead we use the similarly golden-hued turmeric, a spice with powerful anti-inflammatory antioxidants.

Preheat the oven to 450°F. Coat a large rimmed baking sheet with cooking spray.

In a large bowl, whisk together 1 tablespoon oil, the vinegar, mustard, smoked paprika, ¼ teaspoon salt, and pepper. Add the cauliflower and toss well. Spread the cauliflower evenly on the baking sheet. Roast for about 20 minutes, until fork-tender.

Meanwhile, heat the remaining 1 tablespoon oil in a large skillet over medium heat. Add the bell pepper and cook, stirring occasionally, until it just starts to soften, 5 minutes. Push the peppers to the outer edges of the skillet. Add the garlic and turmeric and cook, stirring constantly, until the garlic just begins to turn golden, about 1 minute. Add the rice and stir until the grains are lightly toasted, for 2 to 3 minutes. Add the broth, tomatoes with their juices, and remaining ¼ teaspoon salt. Turn the heat to high and bring to a boil. Cover, reduce the heat to medium, and cook until the rice is tender, about 10 minutes. Stir in the roasted cauliflower, frozen peas, olives, and reserved olive liquid and heat until the peas are warm, 1 to 2 minutes. Serve with the lemon wedges for squeezing.

PER SERVING: Calories: 408, Total Fat: 12g; Saturated Fat: 2g; Cholesterol: 0mg; Sodium: 834mg; Total Carbohydrates: 70g; Fiber: 10g; Protein: 12g

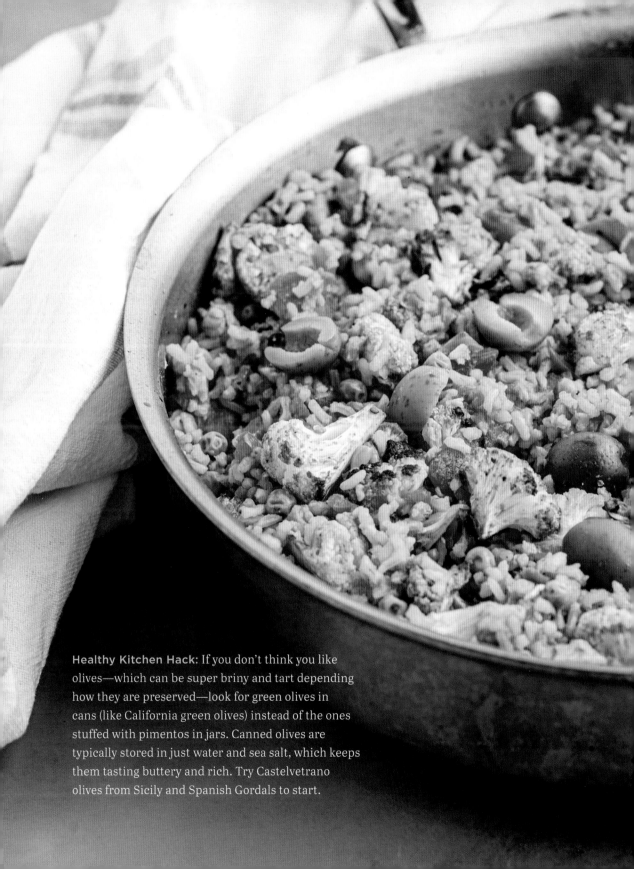

Healthy Kitchen Hack: If you don't think you like olives—which can be super briny and tart depending how they are preserved—look for green olives in cans (like California green olives) instead of the ones stuffed with pimentos in jars. Canned olives are typically stored in just water and sea salt, which keeps them tasting buttery and rich. Try Castelvetrano olives from Sicily and Spanish Gordals to start.

Artichoke Rainbow VEGGIE BAKE

SERVES 6 Prep time: 15 minutes ✻ Cook time: 30 minutes

1 tablespoon extra-virgin olive oil

2 carrots, scrubbed and diced

1 onion, diced

2 garlic cloves, minced

2 (14-ounce) cans artichoke hearts, drained, rinsed, and chopped

1 (12-ounce) jar roasted red peppers, drained, rinsed, and chopped

⅔ cup panko bread crumbs, divided

½ cup chopped fresh parsley leaves and stems

1½ cups shredded part-skim mozzarella

1 cup 2% milk

2 large eggs

¼ teaspoon black pepper

2 tablespoons grated Parmesan cheese

½ teaspoon dried thyme

Abundant in Mediterranean recipes, artichokes are sometimes overlooked in the US, and we think they are a terrific veggie ingredient to include in your routine cooking. They're also loaded with prebiotic fiber plus specific antioxidants that have possible ties to improving memory and mood. Serve this vibrantly colored dish with crusty or multigrain bread as an entrée or in smaller portions as a yummy veggie side.

Preheat the oven to 400° F. Coat a 9 × 13-inch baking pan with cooking spray.

In a medium pot, heat the olive oil over medium heat. Add the carrots and onion and cook, stirring occasionally, until they just start to soften, about 5 minutes. Add the garlic and cook, stirring frequently, until fragrant, 1 minute. Remove from the heat and mix in the artichokes and roasted peppers. Transfer the mix to the prepared baking pan. Stir in ⅓ cup panko and the parsley.

In a separate bowl, whisk together the mozzarella, milk, eggs, and black pepper. Pour over the ingredients in the baking pan and gently mix everything together.

In a small bowl, mix the remaining ⅓ cup panko, Parmesan cheese, and thyme. Sprinkle over the top of the veggie mix. Bake for 20 to 25 minutes, until the center is just set. Remove from the oven and let sit for 10 minutes (it will continue to set), then cut into 6 large slices or 12 small slices to serve.

Healthy Kitchen Hack: If you want to reduce the sodium in this recipe further (besides draining and rinsing the jarred goods), look for frozen artichoke hearts at your market to replace the canned ones. You can also swap in a chopped large bell pepper for the jarred peppers and cook it with the onion and carrots.

PER SERVING: Calories: 272; Total Fat: 12g; Saturated Fat: 6g; Cholesterol: 89mg; Sodium: 693mg; Total Carbohydrates: 28g; Fiber: 4g; Protein: 14g

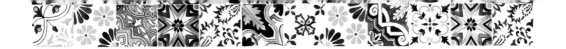

GREEN FALAFEL FRITTERS
with Red Pepper Sauce

SERVES 4   Prep time: 20 minutes   ❋   Cook time: 35 minutes

Throughout the Middle East, there may be as many versions of falafel as there are street vendors who sell them. Our fresh take is a gorgeous green chickpea fritter served with a bright and nutty red pepper sauce. The almonds in the sauce are rich in healthy fats, which help keep blood flowing efficiently to the brain. Frozen green peas add fiber and bright color appeal to falafel, which are often a monochromatic brown; the green hue alone had Serena's family loving these fritters even before they tasted them.

Heat 1 tablespoon oil in a large skillet over medium heat. Add the scallions and cook, stirring occasionally, until they begin to soften, 4 minutes. Add the garlic and cook, stirring constantly, until fragrant, about 1 minute. Remove from the heat and transfer half of the vegetables to a food processor.

Using a Microplane or citrus zester, grate the zest from the lemon into the food processor, then cut the lemon in half and squeeze in about 1½ tablespoons lemon juice from one half (reserve the other half for the falafel).

To the food processor, add the red peppers and 3 tablespoons reserved red pepper liquid, almonds, and ¼ teaspoon salt. Start to pulse while slowly drizzling in 2 tablespoons oil—the sauce should be semi-thick and textured. (For a thinner sauce, drizzle in more red pepper liquid.) Transfer the sauce to a serving bowl and set aside.

continued on page 157

4 tablespoons extra-virgin olive oil, divided

6 scallions (green onions), green and white parts, chopped

3 garlic cloves, minced

1 lemon

1 (12-ounce) jar roasted red peppers, drained (liquid reserved)

½ cup chopped almonds

½ teaspoon kosher or sea salt, divided

1½ cups frozen peas, thawed

⅓ cup whole-wheat bread crumbs (about 1 slice of toast, crumbled)

¼ cup whole-wheat or all-purpose flour

1 cup chopped fresh cilantro, parsley, and/or mint leaves and stems

1 teaspoon ground cumin

½ teaspoon black pepper

¾ cup hummus (see Hack)

⅓ cup crumbled feta cheese

4 cups baby spinach or other leafy greens

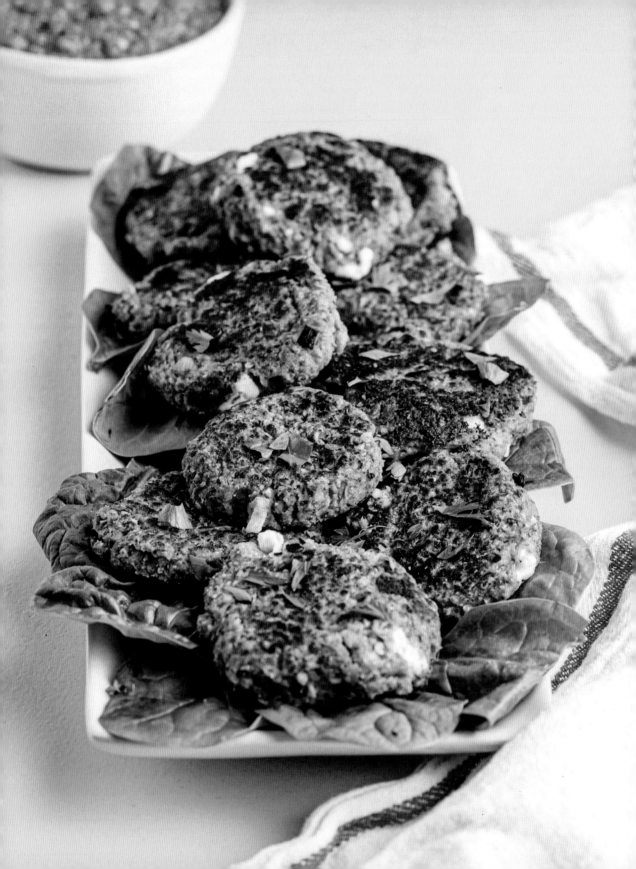

continued from page 155

To the food processor (no need to clean), add the remaining cooked scallion mixture, peas, bread crumbs, flour, herbs, cumin, black pepper, and remaining ¼ teaspoon salt, then squeeze in the juice from the reserved lemon half. Pulse about 10 times, until the mixture is combined but still has some texture. Add the hummus and pulse 5 to 7 times, until the hummus is incorporated throughout. Transfer the mixture to a medium bowl and stir in the cheese.

Using a 1½-tablespoon cookie scoop or measuring spoon, shape the mixture into portions about the size of a walnut and place on a plate; you should get about 20.

Heat the remaining 1 tablespoon oil in the same skillet over medium heat. Add 7 falafel balls and, using a fork, flatten each to a ½-inch thickness. Cook until golden brown and crispy on the outside, 8 to 10 minutes, flipping halfway through. Transfer to a serving plate and cover to keep warm while cooking the remaining falafel in 2 more batches.

Scatter the leafy greens on a large platter and top with the falafel balls. Serve with the red pepper sauce on the side for dipping or drizzling.

Healthy Kitchen Hack: If you aren't convinced yet that making hummus is worth it, hopefully this recipe gets you into the habit, because homemade is so, so good! In a food processor or high-powered blender, blend 1 (15-ounce) can chickpeas, drained (liquid reserved) and rinsed, plus ¼ cup of the chickpea liquid, 2 tablespoons peanut butter or tahini, and ¼ teaspoon kosher or sea salt. With the blender on, drizzle in 2 tablespoons extra-virgin olive oil and process until smooth, adding more chickpea liquid or water for the desired texture.

PER SERVING: Calories: 458; Total Fat: 31g; Saturated Fat: 5g; Cholesterol: 11mg; Sodium: 616mg; Total Carbohydrates: 36g; Fiber: 9g; Protein: 14g

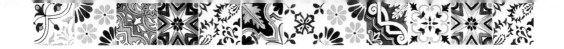

One-Pot
SPANISH BEANS AND BARLEY

SERVES 6 Prep time: 20 minutes ✳ Cook time: 30 minutes

2 tablespoons extra-virgin olive oil

1 onion, chopped

1 bell pepper (any color), seeded and chopped

1 jalapeño pepper, seeded and chopped (optional)

3 garlic cloves, minced

2 teaspoons smoked paprika or 1 tablespoon chili powder

½ teaspoon black pepper

1 cup quick pearl barley

Leaves from 2 thyme sprigs or 1 teaspoon dried thyme

½ teaspoon kosher or sea salt

2 (15-ounce) cans great northern beans or other white beans, drained and rinsed (see Hack)

1 (14.5-ounce) can low-sodium fire-roasted or regular diced tomatoes, undrained

1 mandarin orange or clementine

½ cup chopped almonds

1 cucumber, chopped

1 tablespoon balsamic vinegar

The list of ingredients for Spain's classic chilled tomato soup gazpacho sounds enticing: bell peppers, onions, garlic, balsamic vinegar, citrus, almonds, smoked paprika, black pepper, and hot chiles, all cooled by fresh tomatoes and cucumbers. But Serena just can't learn to love the idea of cold soup. So she created a warm and comforting dish using the flavors of gazpacho to complement a pot of beans and grains—a true staple combination around the Mediterranean. In Spain, fiber- and nutrient-rich barley is the primary grain crop. Also, tomatoes contain lycopene, a powerful bioactive compound that may reduce some oxidative damage in the brain. Lycopene is more easily absorbed from cooked tomatoes—just another reason Serena prefers this warm spiced tomato dish to cold gazpacho.

Heat the oil in a Dutch oven or large stockpot over medium heat. Add the onion, bell pepper, and jalapeño (if using) and cook, stirring occasionally, until they begin to soften, 8 to 10 minutes. Add the garlic, smoked paprika, and black pepper and cook, stirring occasionally, until fragrant, 1 minute. Add the barley, thyme, salt, and 3 cups water and bring to a boil. Turn the heat to medium-low, cover, and simmer for 10 to 12 minutes, until the barley is tender. Add the beans, tomatoes with their juices, and ½ cup water (from rinsing out the tomato can) and add to the pot. Heat until warm, about 5 minutes, stirring occasionally.

While the barley cooks, using a Microplane or citrus zester, grate the zest from the orange into a small bowl, then cut the orange in half and squeeze in the juice.

When the barley and beans are heated through, stir in the orange zest, orange juice, and almonds and heat through. Ladle into bowls, top with the cucumber and balsamic vinegar, and serve.

Healthy Kitchen Hack: Swap in a 1-pound bag of dried great northern beans for the canned beans. Soak the beans in a Dutch oven or large pot in 8 cups water for at least 6 hours or overnight. Drain the soaking water, add 6 cups fresh water, 1 quartered onion, and 1 teaspoon kosher or sea salt, and bring to a boil over high heat. Turn the heat to low and simmer with the lid vented for about 1 hour, until the beans are tender (occasionally checking to make sure there is still plenty of liquid in the pot to prevent scorching). Use any remaining liquid in the bean pot in place of the water in this recipe, or in other soup recipes.

PER SERVING: Calories: 362; Total Fat: 9g; Saturated Fat: 1g; Cholesterol: 0mg; Sodium: 508mg; Total Carbohydrates: 59g; Fiber: 14g; Protein: 15g

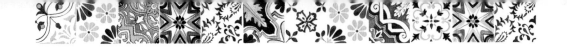

RATATOUILLE *with Socca*

SERVES 6 Prep time: 20 minutes ✳ Cook time: 50 minutes

1 cup chickpea
(garbanzo bean) flour

10 tablespoons extra-virgin
olive oil, divided

½ teaspoon kosher
or sea salt, divided

½ teaspoon black pepper,
divided

1 large onion, chopped

1 bell pepper
(red, orange, or yellow),
seeded and chopped

1 large zucchini, unpeeled,
cut into ¾-inch cubes

1 small eggplant, unpeeled,
cut into ¾-inch cubes

4 garlic cloves, minced

4 large tomatoes, seeded
and coarsely chopped

1 teaspoon sugar
(optional)

3 thyme sprigs

1 bay leaf (optional)

6 fresh basil leaves, torn

Wendy, the owner of Bliss Travels and the designer of our Mediterranean culinary trips, says the secret to a great ratatouille is to cook each vegetable separately for the most tantalizing flavor. Most Provençal families have their own recipe, and you too can modify this one to your liking (or with what you have on hand). We serve the veggie stew with another South of France staple, socca—the delicious chickpea pancake/flatbread. You'll get a hefty dose of monounsaturated fats from the olive oil and antioxidants and fiber from the veggies—all important natural plant nutrients that can protect our brain and mental health.

To make the socca batter, in a large bowl, whisk together the chickpea flour, 2 tablespoons oil, ¼ teaspoon salt, and ¼ teaspoon black pepper. Continue to whisk while slowly pouring in ¾ cup water until a thin batter forms. Set aside while you make the ratatouille, to allow the flour to absorb the water.

In a large pot or a Dutch oven, heat 1 tablespoon oil over medium heat. Add the onions and cook, stirring occasionally, until lightly browned, about 5 minutes. Add the bell pepper and cook, stirring occasionally, until tender-crisp, about 3 minutes. Transfer to a colander (so any moisture drains out for the most concentrated flavors), wipe out the pan, and return it to the stove.

Add 2 tablespoons oil and reheat the pan. Add the zucchini and cook, stirring occasionally, until slightly wilted, 4 to 5 minutes. Transfer to the colander, wipe out the pan, and return it to the stove.

Add another 2 tablespoons oil and reheat the pan. Add the eggplant and cook, stirring occasionally, until slightly wilted, 4 to 5 minutes. Transfer to the colander, wipe out the pan, and return it to the stove.

continued on page 162

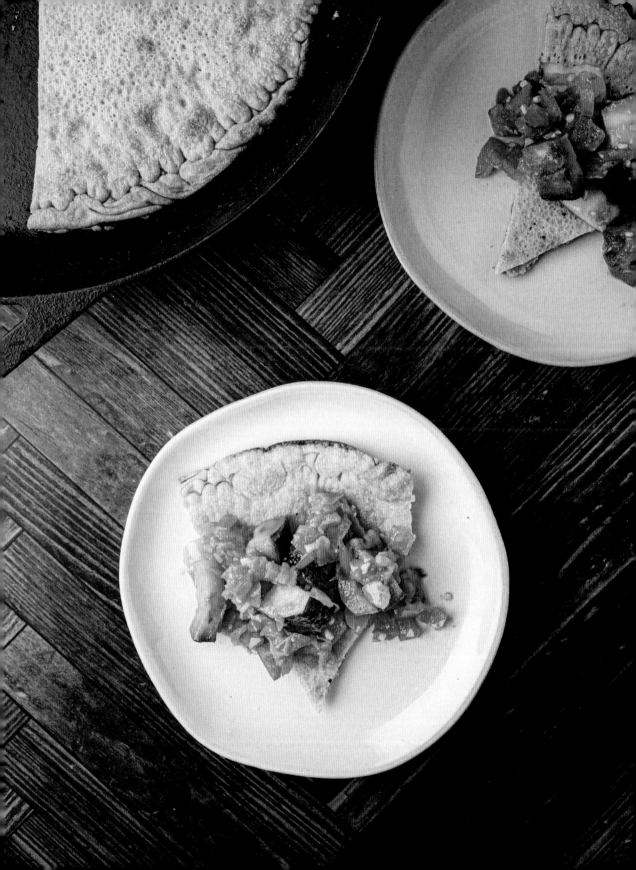

continued from page 160

Add another 1 tablespoon oil and reheat the pan. Add the garlic and cook, stirring frequently, for 30 seconds. Add the tomatoes, sugar (if you have very ripe tomatoes, the sugar is unnecessary), thyme sprigs, and bay leaf, if using. Bring to a boil. Add the previously cooked vegetables, remaining ¼ teaspoon salt, and remaining ¼ teaspoon black pepper. Stir well and reduce the heat to medium-low. Cover and cook, stirring occasionally, for about 30 minutes, until the vegetables are very tender. Turn off the heat and discard the thyme sprigs and bay leaf, if used. Stir in the basil.

While the ratatouille cooks, place the top oven rack about 6 inches below the broiler element. Pour 1 tablespoon oil into a large cast-iron skillet. Place the skillet in the oven and preheat the oven to 450°F.

When the oven is hot and the vegetables are done, carefully remove the skillet from the oven, swirl around the hot oil, and then pour the socca batter into the skillet. Tilt the skillet until the batter is evenly spread out. Bake until the edges are golden brown and the center is dry, 12 to 14 minutes. Remove the skillet from the oven and turn on the broiler.

Brush the socca with the remaining 1 tablespoon oil, then broil for 1½ minutes, or until the top has some golden brown spots (be careful not to burn the edges). Remove from the oven and cut into 6 wedges.

To serve, place a socca wedge on each plate and top with about ½ cup ratatouille. You will have extra ratatouille, which will keep in an airtight container in the refrigerator for up to 5 days. (It will taste even more delicious the next day, whether cold or reheated!)

Healthy Kitchen Hack: Here are a few optional swaps in a pinch: instead of fresh tomatoes, use 1 (14.5-ounce) can diced tomatoes with their juices; instead of bell pepper, use ½ (12-ounce) jar chopped roasted red peppers in their liquid; instead of thyme sprigs, use ½ teaspoon dried thyme or herbes de Provence.

PER SERVING: Calories: 353; Total Fat: 25g; Saturated Fat: 4g; Cholesterol: 0mg; Sodium: 188mg; Total Carbohydrates: 30g; Fiber: 7g; Protein: 7g

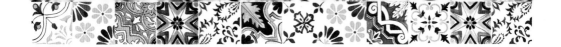

7-Spice
MUSHROOM BULGUR STUFFED ZUCCHINI

SERVES 4 Prep time: 15 minutes ✴ Cook time: 30 minutes

The flavors of this satisfying vegetarian entrée are inspired by the aromatic Lebanese 7-spice blend sabaa baharat, which commonly features a base of ground cumin, cinnamon, cloves, and black pepper, plus a few more spices depending on the region, manufacturer, or family preference. Tomato bulgur pilaf is a common dish in Lebanon. With the addition of mushrooms, this is a super smart veggie-packed dish for your brain and mood!

Cut the ends off each zucchini and then cut in half lengthwise so you have eight halves. Using a teaspoon, scoop out the center of each zucchini half, leaving a ½-inch shell (to create a vessel for the stuffing). Finely chop the scooped-out parts and set aside.

In a large Dutch oven or saucepan, heat 2 tablespoons oil over medium heat. Add the onion and cook, stirring frequently, until just beginning to soften, 3 minutes. Add the garlic and cook, stirring frequently, until fragrant, 1 minute. Add the mushrooms and chopped zucchini and cook, stirring frequently, until beginning to soften, 5 minutes. Add the bulgur, cumin, cinnamon, coriander, nutmeg, salt, pepper, and cloves and cook, stirring frequently, for 2 minutes. Stir in 2 cups water and the tomato paste until the ingredients are incorporated, then bring to a boil. Reduce the heat to low, stir, cover, and cook for 10 minutes. Stir again, cover, and cook for another 5 minutes, or until all the liquid is absorbed. Remove from the heat. Using a Microplane or citrus zester, grate the zest from the lemon into the pot, then cut the lemon in half and squeeze in the juice. Mix and fluff with a fork, then cover to keep warm until serving.

4 medium zucchini

3 tablespoons extra-virgin olive oil, divided

½ onion, finely chopped

2 garlic cloves, minced

8 ounces mushrooms (such as button, cremini, and/or others), finely chopped

1 cup bulgur

½ teaspoon ground cumin

¼ teaspoon ground cinnamon

¼ teaspoon ground coriander

¼ teaspoon ground nutmeg

¼ teaspoon kosher or sea salt

¼ teaspoon black pepper

⅛ teaspoon ground cloves

3 tablespoons tomato paste

1 lemon

½ cup plain whole-milk Greek yogurt or Homemade Yogurt (page 60)

continued on page 165

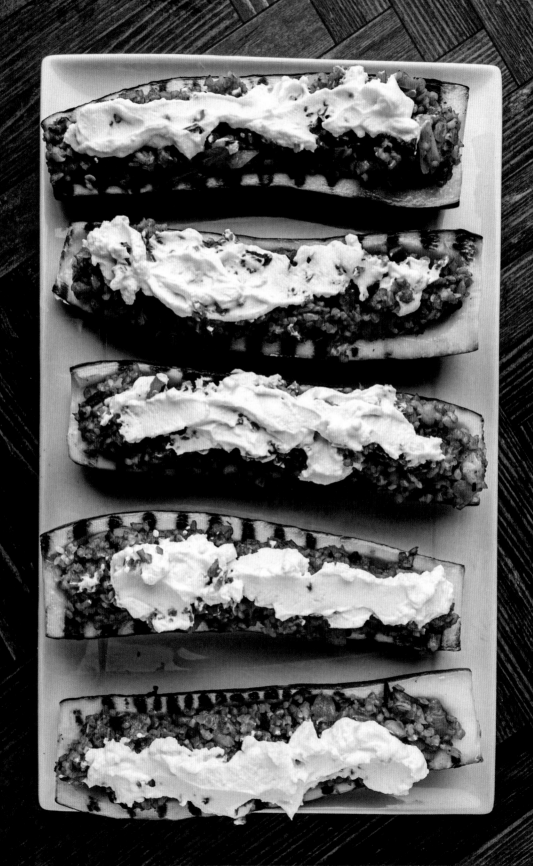

continued from page 163

While the bulgur cooks, preheat an outdoor grill to 400°F or a stovetop grill pan over medium-high heat. Brush the cut side of each zucchini half with the remaining 1 tablespoon oil. Working in batches if necessary, place the zucchini halves on the grill or grill pan, cut side down, and grill for 3 to 5 minutes, until slightly golden and charred underneath. Flip and cook for an additional 3 to 5 minutes, until the zucchini has softened and is just cooked through. Transfer the zucchini to a serving platter. Into each half, spoon about ⅔ cup of the bulgur stuffing (you will not use all the stuffing—see the Hack). Top each half with a dollop of yogurt and serve immediately.

Tip: The cool, creamy yogurt spooned on top of this dish adds a lovely contrast to the 7 spices, but if you want to make this dish vegan, simply skip it.

Healthy Kitchen Hack: The bonus with this recipe is the leftover stuffing that will keep in an airtight container in the refrigerator for up to 3 days. Reheat and serve as a side dish, or mix with spinach or arugula for a cold grain and greens salad, or toss with scrambled eggs for a protein-packed breakfast. Or try stuffing into other hollowed-out grilled veggies, like large tomatoes, portobello mushrooms, eggplant halves, or bell peppers.

PER SERVING: (2 zucchini halves): Calories: 341; Total Fat: 14g; Saturated Fat: 3g; Cholesterol: 5mg; Sodium: 177mg; Total Carbohydrates: 47g; Fiber: 10g; Protein: 14g

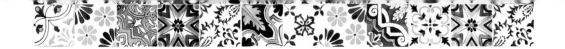

MUSHROOM DAUBE

SERVES 6   Prep time: 25 minutes   ✳ Cook time: 50 minutes

1 small orange or
mandarin orange

2 tablespoons extra-virgin
olive oil

3 carrots, scrubbed and
cut into ¼-inch rounds

2 leeks, white, light green,
and some dark green
parts, thinly sliced

1 large onion, diced

3 garlic cloves, minced

1½ pounds mushrooms
(such as button, cremini,
and/or others), thickly
sliced

½ teaspoon kosher
or sea salt

¼ teaspoon black pepper

1 pound red potatoes
(about 4 medium),
scrubbed and cut into
¼-inch pieces

3 tablespoons
all-purpose flour

2 cups low-sodium
vegetable broth

3 thyme sprigs or
1 teaspoon dried thyme

2 rosemary sprigs or
1 teaspoon dried rosemary

2 bay leaves

1 cup dry red wine

2 tablespoons
tomato paste

1 tablespoon
less-sodium soy sauce

Daube is the quintessential Provençal meat stew featuring beef, vegetables, and herbs braised in a red wine sauce. The saying goes there are as many versions of daube as there are cooks in France. Our vegetarian version highlights one of our favorite brain boosters: the mighty mushroom. We also use a secret ingredient—soy sauce—to kick up the savory flavor that typically comes from beef. Serve it one of many ways that French cooks do, like over mashed potatoes, polenta, or wide noodles, or simply enjoy right out of the bowl with baguette slices for sopping up the sauce.

Using a vegetable peeler, peel off two 3-inch strips of orange rind and set aside (save the remaining orange for another use).

In a large Dutch oven or stockpot, heat the olive oil over medium heat. Add the carrots, leeks, and onion and cook, stirring occasionally, until slightly softened, 5 minutes. Add the garlic and cook, stirring frequently, for 1 minute. Stir in the mushrooms, salt, and black pepper, cover, and cook, stirring a few times, until softened, 10 minutes. Stir in the potatoes and flour until well incorporated and cook for 1 minute. Stir in the broth, scraping the sides and bottom of the pot to incorporate the flour mixture. Simmer until the stew just starts to boil, then stir, reduce the heat to medium-low, and add the orange rinds, thyme, rosemary, and bay leaves. Let simmer, stirring occasionally and scraping the bottom of the pot, for 15 minutes, or until the potatoes are cooked through.

Stir in the wine, tomato paste, and soy sauce. Return to a simmer and cook, stirring occasionally and scraping the bottom of the pot, for at least another 15 minutes, until the stew is thick and the vegetables are soft (the longer it simmers, the thicker and more flavorful the stew will become). Before serving, remove the orange peels, thyme sprigs, rosemary sprigs, and bay leaves.

Healthy Kitchen Hack: For an extra nod to the south of France, tinker with your daube recipe by adding olives or capers. Spice it up with 1 teaspoon ground cinnamon and ¼ teaspoon ground cloves or with 2 teaspoons herbes de Provence. Or stir in ½ cup chopped prunes for a hint of sweetness.

66

I'm not a mushroom fan, but this tasted like beef stew to me!

LEO FROM WEST CHESTER, PA

PER SERVING: Calories: 225; Total Fat: 6g; Saturated Fat: 1g; Cholesterol: 0mg; Sodium: 331mg; Total Carbohydrates: 33g; Fiber: 6g; Protein: 7g

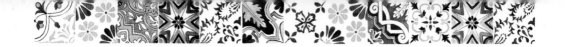

CRISP CORN CAKES
with Goat Cheese and Tomatoes

SERVES 4 (makes 16 corn cakes) Prep time: 20 minutes ✳ Cook time: 15 minutes

½ cup white whole-wheat, whole-wheat, or all-purpose flour

½ cup cornmeal

1 teaspoon baking powder

½ teaspoon black pepper

¼ teaspoon kosher or sea salt

⅛ teaspoon crushed red pepper

2 large eggs

⅓ cup 2% milk

1 cup frozen corn kernels, thawed

½ cup chopped fresh or low-sodium canned tomatoes, undrained

⅓ cup crumbled goat cheese

1 teaspoon fresh thyme leaves or ½ teaspoon dried thyme, plus more for garnish (optional)

4 tablespoons extra-virgin olive oil, divided

1 lemon, cut into wedges

What's better than sitting down to a stack of fluffy corn cakes? Serena's dinner guests (her kids and grandma) were pretty excited until they found out there was no maple syrup. But when they tasted them with another topping they adore—brain-boosting, antioxidant-rich olives—they gave rave reviews. If you're an olive lover like the Ball kids, try these topped with the Green Olive Salsa Verde from our Roasted Radishes (page 89). Or try other favorite condiments like hot sauce, honey, or yogurt. Or simply enjoy them as is, with a squeeze of lemon juice.

In a large bowl, whisk together the flour, cornmeal, baking powder, black pepper, salt, and crushed red pepper. In a medium bowl, whisk together the eggs and milk, then stir in the corn, tomatoes with their juices, goat cheese, and thyme. Pour over the flour mixture and stir just to combine; don't overmix. Let sit for 10 minutes for the flour mixture to hydrate. Meanwhile, preheat the oven or toaster oven to 200°F.

Heat 1 tablespoon oil in a large skillet over medium heat. Spoon about 2 tablespoons batter per corn cake into the skillet; cook in batches of four to avoid crowding. Cook until bubbles on the top begin to pop (similar to a pancake) and brown on the bottom, about 2 minutes. Flip the cakes and cook until brown on the other side, an additional 1 to 2 minutes. Transfer to a rimmed baking sheet and keep warm in the oven. Repeat cooking in batches with the remaining batter and 1 tablespoon oil per batch, for a total of 16 corn cakes. Garnish with extra thyme, if desired, and serve warm with lemon wedges for squeezing.

PER SERVING: Calories: 338; Total Fat: 20g; Saturated Fat: 5g; Cholesterol: 99mg; Sodium: 251mg; Total Carbohydrates: 33g; Fiber: 4g; Protein: 10g

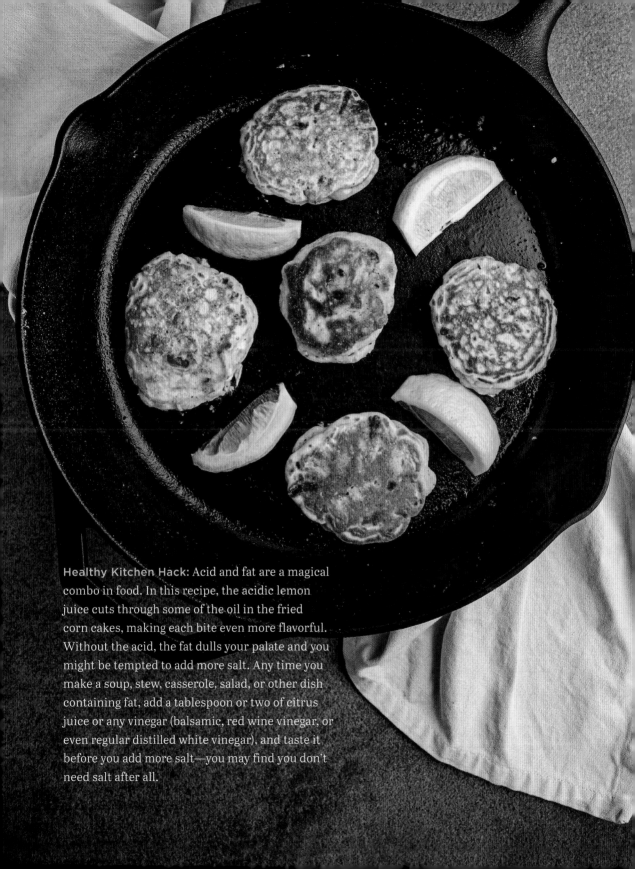

Healthy Kitchen Hack: Acid and fat are a magical combo in food. In this recipe, the acidic lemon juice cuts through some of the oil in the fried corn cakes, making each bite even more flavorful. Without the acid, the fat dulls your palate and you might be tempted to add more salt. Any time you make a soup, stew, casserole, salad, or other dish containing fat, add a tablespoon or two of citrus juice or any vinegar (balsamic, red wine vinegar, or even regular distilled white vinegar), and taste it before you add more salt—you may find you don't need salt after all.

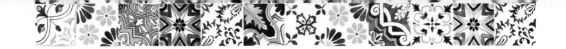

EGYPTIAN KOSHARI
with Sautéed Onions

SERVES 4 Prep time: 15 minutes ✳ Cook time: 45 minutes

1 lime

4 tablespoons extra-virgin olive oil, divided

2 onions, thinly sliced (see Hack)

½ cup brown lentils

½ cup instant brown rice

½ cup elbow pasta

½ teaspoon kosher or sea salt

2 garlic cloves, minced

½ teaspoon black pepper

½ teaspoon ground cumin

½ teaspoon ground coriander

⅛–¼ teaspoon crushed red pepper

1 (14.5-ounce) can low-sodium diced tomatoes, undrained

Known as the national dish of Egypt, koshari is a street food favorite consisting of various combinations of legumes, rice, and pasta all topped with a zesty tomato sauce and golden fried onions. Like many global cuisines, the Mediterranean diet is fueled by carbohydrates, mainly from nutrient-rich pasta, rice, lentils, beans, and starchy veggies. Our brains rely on carbs for fuel. Plus, eating carbs that also contain protein at the evening meal aids in serotonin production in the brain, which helps induce sleep. And sleep is essential for the body's rest and repair from head to toe.

Using a Microplane or citrus zester, grate the zest from the lime into a small bowl, then cut the lime in half and squeeze in 1 tablespoon juice. Squeeze another 1 tablespoon lime juice into another small bowl. Set both bowls aside.

Heat 3 tablespoons oil in a Dutch oven or large saucepan over medium heat. Add the onions and cook, stirring occasionally, for 15 to 20 minutes, until golden brown. Transfer the onions to a plate and set aside (do not wipe out the pot). Add the lentils and 3 cups water to the pot and bring to a boil over high heat. Cover, reduce the heat to medium-low, and cook for 8 minutes. Turn the heat back up to medium and stir in the rice. Cover the pot and cook for 7 minutes, then stir in the pasta, cover again, and cook until the liquid is mostly absorbed and the pasta is al dente, about 8 more minutes. Remove the pot from the heat and let it sit, covered, for 1 minute. Stir in the salt and the 1 tablespoon lime juice with the lime zest.

While the lentils cook, heat the remaining 1 tablespoon oil in a medium saucepan over medium heat. Add the garlic, black pepper, cumin, coriander, and red pepper and cook, stirring frequently, for 1 minute, or until fragrant. Pour in the tomatoes with their juices, stir, and cook for about 10 minutes, until slightly thickened. Stir in the reserved 1 tablespoon lime juice. Add about one-third of the sautéed onions, then transfer the mixture to a food processor or blender. Process until smooth, then pour the mixture into a serving bowl.

Divide the koshari rice mixture among 4 bowls and serve with the tomato sauce and remaining sautéed onions alongside for toppings.

Tip: Yes, you'll have two pots going for the base and the sauce, but you'll be cooking up a whole lot of comfort food heaven. So, while you're at it, make a double batch of this recipe to enjoy for later—it's just as good or even better the next day, heated or at room temperature.

Healthy Kitchen Hack: It may seem daunting to slice two onions (about 3 cups) and then cook them for 20 minutes— or, if you double this recipe, 6 cups for 30 minutes. Here are two tips to help: (1) Use the food processor's slicing attachment (not the chopper) to slice all the onions in seconds and (2) use the slow cooker to cook up a bigger batch of caramelized onions ahead of time—or even to store in the fridge for topping pizza, baked potatoes (see page 174), pasta/rice/beans, and roasted vegetables. Coat a slow cooker with cooking spray, add 2 pounds (about 8 cups) thinly sliced onions, 2 tablespoons extra-virgin olive oil, and ½ teaspoon kosher or sea salt. Mix, cover, and cook on high for 4 hours or on low for 6 to 8 hours without stirring.

66
I liked eating lentils, rice, and pasta all in the same dish, so much so that I ate it the next morning for breakfast with an egg on top. Next time I'll add more garlic and some bright green parsley.

KIM FROM
PALM DESERT, CA

PER SERVING: Calories: 383; Total Fat: 15g; Saturated Fat: 2g; Cholesterol: 0mg; Sodium: 319mg; Total Carbohydrates: 54g; Fiber: 7g; Protein: 11g

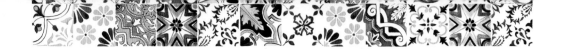

Potato and Cheese
BOUREKAS

SERVES 4 Prep time: 20 minutes ✳ Cook time: 30 minutes

1 small russet potato, scrubbed and cut into ½-inch cubes

¼ cup crumbled feta cheese

¼ cup whole-milk ricotta

1 tablespoon extra-virgin olive oil

1 garlic clove, minced

¼ teaspoon kosher or sea salt

¼ teaspoon black pepper

1 refrigerated pie dough for a 9-inch pie, at room temperature

1 large egg white

1 teaspoon sesame seeds

1 cup jarred tomato sauce or leftover tomato sauce from Egyptian Koshari with Sautéed Onions (page 170)

66

The flaky crust topped with toasted sesame seeds was my favorite part. I also really liked dipping them in the sauce.

JENNIFER FROM
ONTARIO, CANADA

When she traveled to Israel, Deanna tasted popular pocket breads called bourekas stuffed with cheese, potato, and spinach. In Turkey, they're called böreks, and our literary agent, Clare, enjoys them stuffed with eggplant, tomatoes, and/or cheese. Cooks around the Levant form these bread pockets into beautiful shapes from spirals to triangles to something like our half-moon pockets.

Preheat the oven to 400°F. Line a large rimmed baking sheet with parchment paper.

Put the potato in a medium microwave-safe bowl, pour in ¼ cup water, cover with a paper towel, and microwave for about 4 minutes, until fork-tender. Mash the potato with any remaining water. Add the feta, ricotta, oil, garlic, salt, and pepper and mix well.

Unroll the pie dough. Using a 3½-inch round mason jar lid or cookie cutter, cut 7 circles from the dough. Remove the excess dough and roll (or pat) into a piece of dough that's as thick as the first 7 rounds, then cut out one more circle. Place a small bowl of water next to the dough. In another small bowl, whisk together the egg white and 1 tablespoon water.

Scoop 2 teaspoons of the potato filling onto one half of a dough circle, about ¾ inch from the edge. Dip your finger in the water and smooth it around half of the dough, then fold the round in half and press the edges to seal well. Use a fork to crimp the edges. Place on the lined baking sheet. Repeat with the remaining 7 pieces of dough and the filling (you'll have extra filling).

Using a pastry brush or your fingers, brush the tops of the bourekas with the egg wash (you'll have extra wash). Sprinkle

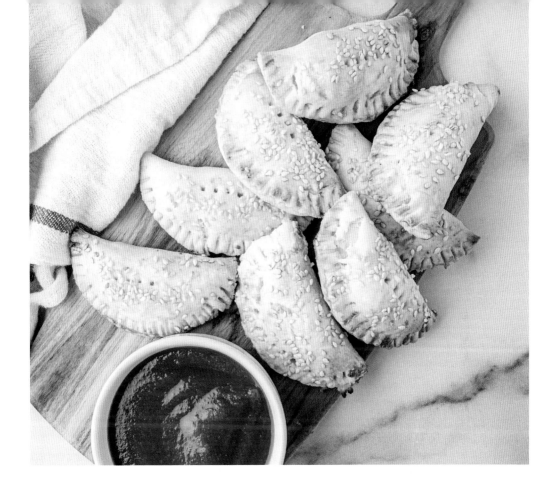

the bourekas with the sesame seeds. Bake for
20 to 25 minutes, until golden. Serve warm with the
tomato sauce.

Tip: Double the recipe to use up the other pie dough that
usually comes in a refrigerated package.

Healthy Kitchen Hack: We love these savory pie-dough
pastries, but they are a bit more authentic when made
with puff pastry—which you can find in the freezer
section of your grocery store. Roll out one sheet of the
thawed pastry dough to ¼-inch thickness and cut into
5-inch squares. Place 1 tablespoon of filling in the center
and fold each corner into the center. Pinch to seal
the edges. Brush with the egg wash and top with sesame
seeds. Bake in a 350°F oven for about 30 minutes,
until golden.

PER SERVING:
(2 bourekas with tomato
sauce): Calories: 353;
Total Fat: 22g; Saturated
Fat: 8g; Cholesterol:
22mg; Sodium: 585mg;
Total Carbohydrates: 36g;
Fiber: 2g; Protein: 6g

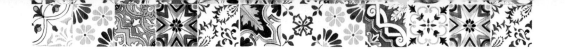

SLOW COOKER BAKED POTATOES
with Mediterranean Toppers

SERVES 6 Prep time: 5 minutes ✳ Cook time: 3 to 6 hours

6 potatoes, well scrubbed (see Hack)

2 teaspoons extra-virgin olive oil

¼ teaspoon kosher or sea salt

Optional Toppings

1 (12-ounce) jar roasted red peppers, drained (liquid saved for another use), finely chopped

1 cup plain 2% Greek yogurt or Homemade Yogurt (page 60)

1 cup crumbled feta or shredded part-skim mozzarella or Manchego cheese

¾ cup chopped sun-dried tomatoes (about 3 ounces), drained if oil-packed (oil saved for another use)

1 (2.25-ounce) can sliced black olives, drained (liquid saved for another use)

Smoked paprika, za'atar, dried oregano, and/or dried thyme

With about 5 minutes of prep time, this veggie main dish may be the easiest recipe in the book. But perhaps you've never heard of "baking" potatoes in your slow cooker? Neither had we until a friend told Serena about this cooking trick. Turns out that slow cooker delivers delectable "baked" potatoes with fluffy insides and crispy skins, especially if you leave them in for a looong time. Enjoy these taters topped with any of our favorite "smart" Mediterranean ingredients below (or from our Eating Smart tips on page 12) or maybe even with leftovers from your fridge!

Pierce the potatoes all over with a fork. In a small bowl, whisk together the oil and salt and then use your fingers to rub the potatoes all over with the mixture.

Place the potatoes in a single layer in a 6- to 7-quart slow cooker. Cover and cook on high for 3 hours or on low for 5 hours (for crispier skins, add 1 to 2 hours to the high or low cooking times). Serve the potatoes warm right out of the crock, with your favorite toppers in small bowls alongside.

Tip: Avoid lifting the lid before 3 hours to check as every time the lid is lifted, 20 minutes must be added to the cooking time!

PER SERVING: Calories: 336; Total Fat: 11g; Saturated Fat: 5g; Cholesterol: 26mg; Sodium: 494mg; Total Carbohydrates: 51g; Fiber: 4g; Protein: 13g (Note: Nutritional values will vary based on toppers.)

Healthy Kitchen Hack:
Slow Cooker Spuds Q&A:

How many? More than 6 potatoes will work as long as they all fit in a single layer in the bottom of the slow cooker. Or do double layers and add about an hour more to your slow cooker times.

What kind? Russet potatoes (aka Idaho potatoes) cook up fluffy like the iconic baked potato. Yukon Gold potatoes cook up moist and creamy. Red potatoes have a firmer, waxier texture but still taste delicious. And sweet potatoes work, too!

What size? The average russet is 2½ inches in diameter and 4 inches long, and will be done in the times specified above. Larger baking potatoes will take about 4 hours on high or 5 to 6 hours on low. Smaller potatoes, like baby golden potatoes, take a minimum of 2½ hours.

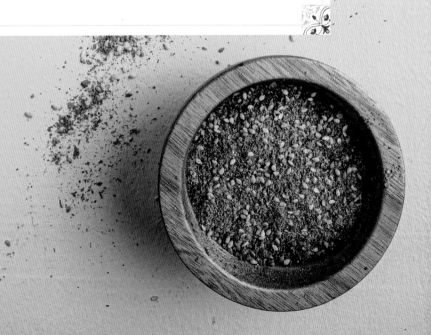

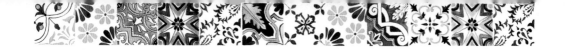

SWEET POTATO FARRO BOWLS *with Pomegranate Molasses*

SERVES 2   Prep time: 20 minutes ❋ Cook time: 25 minutes

½ cup farro or pearl barley

1 medium sweet potato, scrubbed and cut into ¾-inch pieces

½ teaspoon kosher or sea salt, divided

2 teaspoons extra-virgin olive oil

1 tablespoon tahini or peanut butter

1 teaspoon honey

1 teaspoon white wine vinegar

3 cups torn greens (such as spinach, lettuces, and/or leafy herbs)

1 red bell pepper or any other type of pepper, seeded and sliced

¼ cup pistachios, peanuts, or other nuts or seeds

1 tablespoon pomegranate molasses (see Hack)

Pomegranate molasses is a bold, tangy, slightly sweet jewel-colored Middle Eastern condiment. It adds pizzazz to marinades and dressings and is delicious when drizzled on toast, plain yogurt, and this colorful salad bowl recipe, which includes the traditional Italian whole grain farro. Bonus: Pomegranate molasses is loaded with beneficial compounds, including antioxidants and B vitamins, like thiamine, which are essential for certain neurotransmitters in the brain. You may need to buy it online if your grocery store doesn't have it. Or you can make it from scratch—we were delighted to find out how easy it is (see the Hack).

Cook the farro according to the package instructions, without salt. Transfer to a large bowl to cool slightly, about 10 minutes.

While the farro cooks, put the sweet potato in a small pot and cover with water by about an inch. Add ¼ teaspoon salt, cover, and bring to a boil. Uncover, reduce the heat to medium, and cook until just fork-tender, 4 to 6 minutes. Drain the potatoes in a colander, then set aside to cool slightly.

In a large bowl, whisk together the oil, tahini, honey, vinegar, and remaining ¼ teaspoon salt. (If using peanut butter, you may need to add 1 tablespoon hot water to help emulsify the sauce.) Add the greens and cooked farro and toss until well coated.

To assemble the salad bowls, divide the farro mixture between two bowls. Divide the cooked sweet potatoes and the bell pepper between the bowls. Sprinkle with the pistachios. Drizzle with the pomegranate molasses and serve.

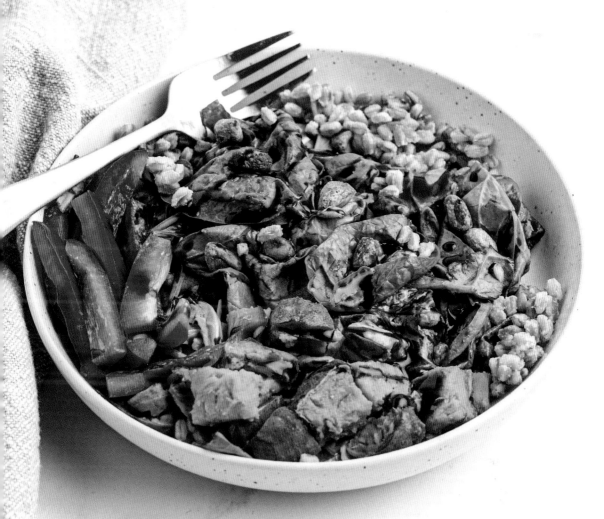

Healthy Kitchen Hack: To make your own pomegranate molasses, whisk together 1 cup pomegranate juice, 2 tablespoons sugar, and 1 teaspoon vinegar (any type) in a small saucepan. Bring to a gentle boil over medium heat. Reduce the heat to medium-low and cook, whisking occasionally, until the liquid is reduced to about ¼ cup and coats the back of a spoon, 30 to 35 minutes. Remove from the stove and let the molasses cool completely. Pour into a glass container, cover, and store in the refrigerator for up to 4 months.

PER SERVING: Calories: 460; Total Fat: 17g; Saturated Fat: 2g; Cholesterol: 0mg; Sodium: 374mg; Total Carbohydrates: 69g; Fiber: 11g; Protein: 14g

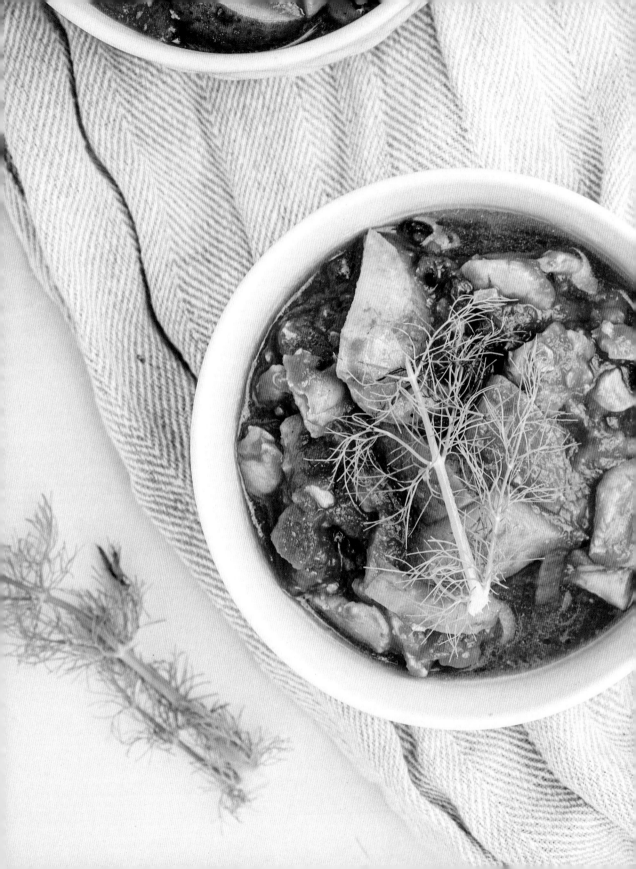

SEAFOOD

QUICK FISH
with Walnut-Arugula Pesto

SERVES 4 Prep time: 10 minutes ✳ Cook time: 5 minutes

1 lemon

2 teaspoons extra-virgin olive oil

4 (4-ounces) tilapia fillets (skin-on or skinless)

¼ teaspoon kosher or sea salt

¼ teaspoon black pepper, divided

½ cup Speedy Pesto Sauce (page 130) made with arugula and walnuts

Healthy Kitchen Hack:
We usually have at least half a lemon tucked away in the fridge, but for the times when the lemon juice "well" is dry, we swap in orange juice, dry white wine, or low-sodium broth for the base cooking liquid in this recipe.

PER SERVING: Calories: 226; Total Fat: 14g; Saturated Fat: 3g; Cholesterol: 59mg; Sodium: 283mg; Total Carbohydrates: 2g; Fiber: 1g; Protein: 24g

We were skeptical when we first heard you could make perfectly cooked fish in the microwave. But we've since become converts, and this method is our number one way to prepare seafood super fast. Mild-flavored tilapia is a great fish for those who aren't big seafood fans and also a good base for the vibrant and intense flavor of this yummy pesto. One serving of tilapia contains 100 percent of the recommended daily value of selenium, a nutrient that has powerful antioxidant properties and is critical for brain health.

Using a Microplane or citrus zester, grate the zest from the lemon into a glass pie dish or large microwave-safe bowl, then cut the lemon in half and squeeze in 2 tablespoons juice (save the remaining lemon for another use). Whisk in the olive oil. Season both sides of the fillets with the salt and pepper. Transfer the fillets to the lemon oil mixture and flip a few times until the fillets are fully coated. With the fillets skin side down (if they have skin), fold each fillet in half crosswise so that all the fillets fit in the dish. Cover the dish with a microwave-safe plate, leaving a small gap at the edge to vent the steam.

Microwave on high for 3 minutes. Carefully remove the hot dish with oven mitts and let some of the steam escape before removing the plate. Check the fillets with a fork to see if the fish is just starting to separate into flakes. If any part doesn't look cooked, cover again and microwave in 15-second increments until done.

Transfer the cooked fish to a serving platter. Spread 2 tablespoons pesto over each fillet.

Pour the sauce from the bottom of the glass dish over the fish and serve.

Easiest BROILED SHRIMP

SERVES 4   Prep time: 5 minutes   ✳   Cook time: 10 minutes

Shrimp are rich in choline, which is linked to proper brain function, including better memory processing. So perhaps you'll remember this quick-fix method for making succulent shrimp—under the broiler! Using shell-on shrimp protects them from drying under the intense heat of the broiler and keeps them plump and super savory. We like to bring the warm baking sheet straight to the table and let everyone grab a few shrimp, shell them, and then dip them in the pan's olive oil juices, along with crusty bread—it's communal and fun!

1 lemon

3 tablespoons extra-virgin olive oil

½ teaspoon garlic powder

½ teaspoon kosher or sea salt

¼ teaspoon crushed red pepper

1 pound frozen shell-on (heads removed) shrimp (31–40 per pound)

Place the top oven rack about 6 inches below the broiler element. Place a large rimmed baking sheet in the oven. Preheat the broiler for at least 10 minutes with the baking sheet inside.

Using a Microplane or citrus zester, grate the zest from the lemon into a large bowl. Cut the lemon into wedges and set aside for serving. To the bowl with the lemon zest, add the oil, garlic powder, salt, and red pepper and mix to combine.

Put the shrimp in a colander and rinse under cold running water for about 1 minute while you break any frozen clumps of shrimp apart and rinse away all ice crystals (but no need to thaw). Shake out the water and transfer the shrimp to a clean towel and blot to remove excess water. Transfer the shrimp to the oil mixture and toss to combine. Carefully remove the hot baking sheet from the oven and pour the shrimp and oil out onto the sheet. Using tongs, spread the shrimp out evenly. Place the sheet back in the oven under the broiler. Broil until the shells begin to get crisp with blistered white spots and the shrimp curl into a C shape and turn opaque, 6 to 8 minutes. (Remember that the shrimp will continue to cook slightly on the hot baking sheet when removed from the oven.)

Serve warm or at room temperature with the lemon wedges for squeezing.

Healthy Kitchen Hack: To make this recipe using fresh or thawed shrimp, broil for only 3 to 5 minutes. You can also use larger shrimp with this technique—21 to 25 shrimp per pound stay plump when broiling; broil for 8 to 10 minutes.

PER SERVING:
(shrimp plus oil on pan):
Calories: 154; Total Fat: 11g;
Saturated Fat: 2g;
Cholesterol: 107mg;
Sodium: 636mg;
Total Carbohydrates: 2g;
Fiber: 0g; Protein: 12g

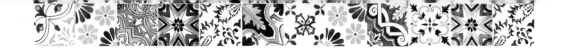

Roasted Salmon and Avocado
FATTOUSH

SERVES 6　Prep time: 15 minutes　✳　Cook time: 15 minutes

1 pound fresh or thawed frozen salmon fillets (skin-on or skinless)

2 avocados, halved and pitted

2 teaspoons honey, divided

¼ teaspoon ground cumin

¼ teaspoon black pepper

2 large whole-wheat pita breads

3 tablespoons extra-virgin olive oil, divided

1 teaspoon za'atar or ½ teaspoon dried thyme plus ½ teaspoon sesame seeds

1 lime

2 cups chopped tomatoes (any kind), divided

½ cup chopped fresh cilantro, divided

1 garlic clove, peeled

¼ teaspoon kosher or sea salt

2 heads romaine lettuce, torn

Fattoush is a traditional salad from northern Lebanon that's also enjoyed in neighboring countries; it features toasted or fried pita, mixed greens, chopped veggies, and lots of fresh herbs. Here we boost this salad's brain benefits with omega-3-rich salmon and monounsaturated fat–loaded avocados—fats that are crucial for cognitive and mental wellness. The creamy, zesty dressing is a riff on fresh salsa and guacamole made "more Mediterranean" with an olive oil base (it's also a delish sandwich spread).

Preheat the oven to 425°F. Line a large rimmed baking sheet with parchment paper.

Arrange the salmon, skin side down (if with skin), and avocado halves, cut sides up, on the lined baking sheet. Drizzle with 1 teaspoon honey and sprinkle with the cumin and black pepper. Bake for 12 to 14 minutes, until the salmon just starts to flake with a fork. Remove from the oven and turn the heat to the broiler setting. Remove the salmon, avocado, and parchment paper from the sheet.

Brush the pitas with 1 tablespoon oil and sprinkle with the za'atar. Place on the same baking sheet and broil until toasted, watching closely to prevent the bread from burning, 1½ to 2 minutes. Cool slightly, then cut or tear into rough 2-inch pieces.

To make the dressing, using a Microplane or citrus zester, grate the zest from the lime into a blender or food processor, then cut the lime in half and squeeze in the juice (save the remaining lime for another use). Scoop the flesh of one of the roasted avocado halves into the blender. Add ½ cup tomatoes, ¼ cup cilantro, the remaining 2 tablespoons oil, remaining 1 teaspoon honey, garlic, salt, and 3 tablespoons

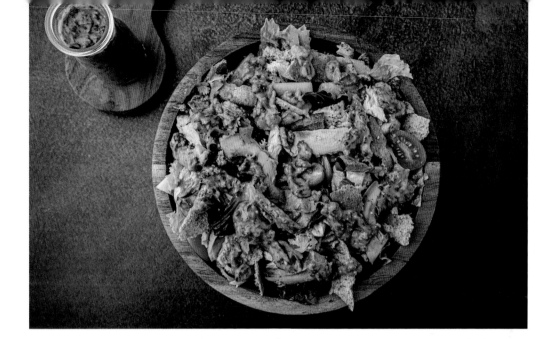

water. Process until a thick but pourable dressing forms. If the dressing seems too thick, add a few more teaspoons of water until it reaches your desired consistency.

When ready to serve, put the lettuce in a serving bowl. Flake the salmon with a fork and add to the lettuce. Holding the flesh side up, cut each remaining avocado half into thin slices (do not cut all the way through the skin). Scoop out the slices with a spoon and add to the salad. Add the remaining 1½ cups tomatoes, remaining ¼ cup cilantro, and the toasted pita pieces. Toss gently, then dollop with about half of the dressing. Serve at room temperature or cold (see Tip) with the remaining dressing on the side.

Tip: If serving the fattoush later or if you want to serve this chilled, refrigerate the various salad ingredients and the dressing separately and toss together right before serving.

Healthy Kitchen Hack: Don't have fresh or frozen salmon on hand for this dish? Then turn to cans! Swap in 1 (16-ounce) can salmon, tuna, mackerel, or any other seafood packed in olive oil to still get the brain benefits of those good fats.

> 66
> *I really liked the texture and variety of flavors in this interesting dish. One option is to skip roasting the avocado and simply use it uncooked.*
>
> TAMMY FROM
> LANGLEY, BC

PER SERVING: Calories: 328; Total Fat: 18g; Saturated Fat: 3g; Cholesterol: 39mg; Sodium: 267mg; Total Carbohydrates: 24g; Fiber: 7g; Protein: 22g

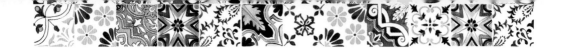

GRILLED FISH
with Almond Honey Mustard Sauce

SERVES 4   Prep time: 15 minutes   ✳   Cook time: 10 minutes

1 pound fresh or thawed frozen Arctic char or salmon fillets (skin-on or skinless), thawed

½ teaspoon black pepper, divided

¼ teaspoon kosher or sea salt

3 tablespoons extra-virgin olive oil, divided

⅓ cup finely chopped almonds

¼ cup Dijon mustard

1 tablespoon honey

2 teaspoons balsamic vinegar

1 teaspoon dried oregano

1 lemon

4 cups salad greens

Seafood brings many cognitive and mental health benefits to the table, but many people are wary about how to cook it. This "no-brainer" recipe will make you a believer in how easy cooking fish on the grill—or a grill pan—can be. It's also "no-brainer" because you won't have to think up a veggie side: the sauce doubles as a scrumptious salad dressing.

Pat the fish dry and let it stand at room temperature for 10 minutes. Meanwhile, coat the cold cooking grate of an outdoor grill with cooking spray, then preheat the grill to 400°F (or heat a stovetop grill pan over medium-high heat).

Sprinkle both sides of the fish evenly with ¼ teaspoon pepper and the salt. Brush both sides with 1 tablespoon olive oil. Carefully lay the fillets on the grill. Close the lid (or cover the grill pan with foil or a large pot lid) and grill until the fish is just opaque, about 10 minutes for each inch of thickness (less time for thinner fillets). Using a wide metal spatula, carefully transfer the fish to a serving platter.

While the fish grills, in a small bowl, whisk together 1 tablespoon oil, the almonds, mustard, honey, vinegar, oregano, and remaining ¼ teaspoon pepper. Pour half of the sauce into a large salad bowl for the dressing (the small bowl will be the sauce for the fish).

Using a Microplane or citrus zester, grate the zest from the lemon into the salad bowl with half of the sauce, then cut the lemon in half and squeeze in 1 tablespoon juice. Cut the remaining lemon half into wedges and set aside for serving. Whisk in the remaining 1 tablespoon oil to achieve a dressing-like consistency. Add the greens and gently toss to coat.

To serve, spread the sauce from the small bowl evenly over the fillets. Serve with the dressed salad and reserved lemon wedges for squeezing.

Tip: For an extra pretty presentation, serve the fish on top of a platter of the dressed greens.

Healthy Kitchen Hack: You can easily switch out some of the ingredients in the sauce with other ingredients in your pantry. Use hazelnuts, peanuts, pecans, pistachios, or walnuts instead of almonds. Dijon mustard is a pungent flavor that is balanced by herbal and cooling herbs like dill, thyme, or tarragon. Mustard is also potent enough to stand up to other strong spices like cumin, onion/garlic powder, or paprika.

PER SERVING: Calories: 328; Total Fat: 20g; Saturated Fat: 3g; Cholesterol: 58mg; Sodium: 561mg; Total Carbohydrates: 9g; Fiber: 2g; Protein: 28g

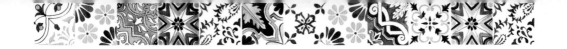

SIZZLING SHRIMP AND PEPPERS *with Cilantro*

SERVES 4 Prep time: 20 minutes ✳ Cook time: 5 minutes

1 pound large shrimp
(31–40 per pound), peeled,
deveined. and patted dry
(see Tip)

½ teaspoon kosher
or sea salt, divided

1 lemon

2 cups chopped fresh
cilantro leaves and stems

3 garlic cloves, sliced,
divided

2 (4-inch) Anaheim
peppers (or 2 jalapeños
for more spice, or 1 large
bell pepper for less spice),
seeded and thinly sliced
into rings, divided

1 teaspoon black pepper

4 tablespoons extra-virgin
olive oil, divided

Even if you have a "low spicy heat" tolerance, you can still get the big brain benefits from hot peppers. Capsaicin is a plant antioxidant found in chiles that delivers powerful anti-inflammatory components for the whole body including the brain. But capsaicin is also found in mildly spicy Anaheim chiles, as well as the spicier jalapeños and spicier yet serranoes. While fresh Mediterranean varieties of hot peppers can be harder to find (although Serena likes to grow varieties like Aleppo or Halaby), use whichever pepper pleases your palate in this simple cilantro shrimp dinner.

In a large bowl, toss the shrimp with ¼ teaspoon salt. Let sit at room temperature for 15 minutes to pull out extra moisture.

Meanwhile, using a Microplane or citrus zester, grate the zest from the lemon into a food processor or high-powered blender, then cut the lemon in half and squeeze in the juice. Add the cilantro, half of the garlic, half of the chiles, the black pepper, and the remaining ¼ teaspoon salt. Process until roughly chopped. Add 1 tablespoon oil and process until smooth.

Heat the remaining 3 tablespoons oil in a large skillet over medium heat. Add the remaining garlic and cook, stirring occasionally, for 1 minute, until fragrant. Reduce the heat to low and stir in the shrimp, the remaining chiles, and the ¼ cup of the cilantro mixture from the blender. Spread the mixture out in an even layer in the skillet, cover with a lid (or baking sheet), and cook for 1 minute without stirring. Uncover and cook, stirring and flipping the shrimp, until they just begin to curl and turn pink opaque on the outside, 1 to 2 minutes. Remove the pan from the heat, cover, and let stand until the shrimp are fully opaque, about 2 minutes. Serve the shrimp with the remaining cilantro mixture.

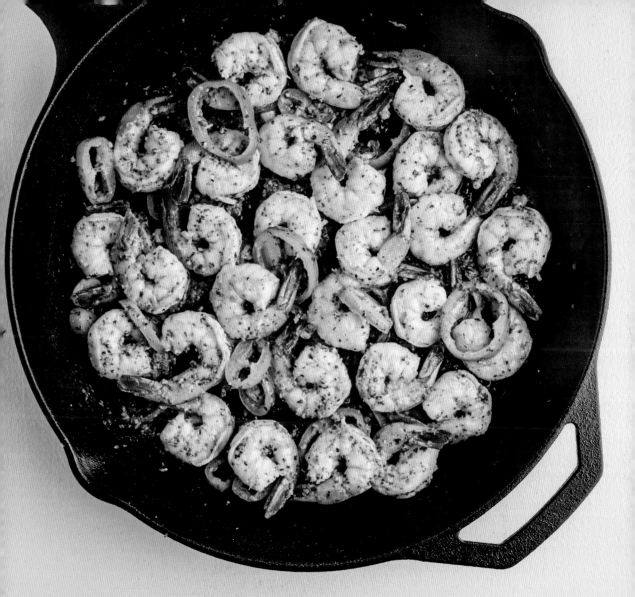

Tip: For the most sustainable choice, look for shrimp from the Pacific Northwest, wild shrimp from the North Atlantic, or USA farmed.

Healthy Kitchen Hack: To avoid overcooking, which results in tough shrimp, we cook them gently over lower heat in a fair amount of oil, which helps buffer the heat. Removing the shrimp from the heat about a minute before they are cooked through also helps, as the residual heat off of the stove will complete the cooking process. This gentle sauté method should yield tender shrimp every time.

PER SERVING: Calories: 238; Total Fat: 15g; Saturated Fat: 2g; Cholesterol: 183mg; Sodium: 432mg; Total Carbohydrates: 5g; Fiber: 1g; Protein: 24g

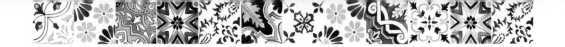

Chermoula
TUNA BURGERS

SERVES 6 Prep time: 15 minutes ✳ Cook time: 25 minutes

¼ teaspoon kosher
or sea salt, divided

½ cup regular or
whole-wheat couscous
(not Israeli couscous)

1 lemon

2 garlic cloves, minced

1 teaspoon
ground coriander

1 teaspoon ground cumin

½ teaspoon
ground turmeric

¼ teaspoon black pepper

¼ teaspoon
cayenne pepper

2 (4.5-ounce) cans
tuna in olive oil, drained
(oil reserved)

⅔ cup plus 2 tablespoons
chopped fresh cilantro
leaves and stems, divided

2 large eggs, lightly beaten

¼ cup plain 2% Greek
yogurt or Homemade
Yogurt (page 60)

2 tablespoons extra-virgin
olive oil, divided

4 cups salad greens
or 4 whole-wheat rolls
(optional)

Chermoula is a pungent condiment popular in Morocco, Algeria, Tunisia, and Libya that's often served with fish. Depending on the region, this spread may have different ingredients, but the base is typically ground coriander, cumin, garlic, lemon, olive oil, and salt. Some versions also have a kick of hot peppers and turmeric, which we really like for color, heat, and of course, the antioxidants that protect our cognitive health. Using the pantry staples of canned tuna (another brain and mood booster) and couscous, it makes whipping up these fish burgers a (Mediterranean) breeze.

Pour ¾ cup water into a medium saucepan and bring to a boil over high heat. Add ⅛ teaspoon salt, then stir in the couscous. Cover, remove from the heat, and allow the couscous to hydrate for 5 minutes. Fluff and then let sit for at least 5 more minutes to cool a bit.

While the couscous cooks, using a Microplane or citrus zester, grate the zest from the lemon into a large bowl, then cut the lemon in half and squeeze in 1 tablespoon lemon juice. Cut the other lemon half into wedges and set aside for serving. To the bowl, add the garlic, coriander, cumin, turmeric, black pepper, cayenne pepper, and remaining ⅛ teaspoon salt and mix well. Transfer half of the spice mix to a small bowl and set aside.

In the large bowl with half of the spices, mix in the cooked couscous and drained tuna. Add ⅔ cup cilantro, the eggs, and yogurt. Gently mix with your hands or a wooden spoon (the mixture will be very wet). Form into 6 patties about 3 inches in diameter and ¾ inch thick.

In a large skillet, heat 1 tablespoon olive oil over medium-high heat. Add 3 patties to the hot oil and reduce the heat to medium. Using a spatula, gently press down on each patty. Cook for 4 minutes until golden brown underneath, then flip the patties and cook for another 3 to 5 minutes, until golden brown. For the second batch, heat the remaining 1 tablespoon olive oil and repeat the cooking process.

While the patties cook, make the chermoula topping. In the small bowl with half of the spice mix, whisk in the reserved oil from the tuna cans (about 1 tablespoon) and the remaining 2 tablespoons cilantro.

Serve the tuna burgers with the reserved lemon wedges for squeezing, either as is, or on top of the salad greens, or inside the rolls. Top each burger with the chermoula sauce.

Healthy Kitchen Hack: Skip the patty shaping and cooking and make "deconstructed" tuna burgers instead! Hydrate 1 cup couscous in 1¼ cups boiling water. Follow the steps above to mix the lemon and spices together and then divide the mixture between two serving bowls. In the first bowl, add the cooked couscous, tuna, and ⅔ cup cilantro (omit the eggs and yogurt) and toss together. In the second bowl, make the chermoula topping as instructed and then toss with 4 cups salad greens. Serve the tuna couscous mix with the dressed salad.

PER SERVING: Calories: 197; Total Fat: 9g; Saturated Fat: 1g; Cholesterol: 78mg; Sodium: 237mg; Total Carbohydrates: 13g; Fiber: 1g; Protein: 16g

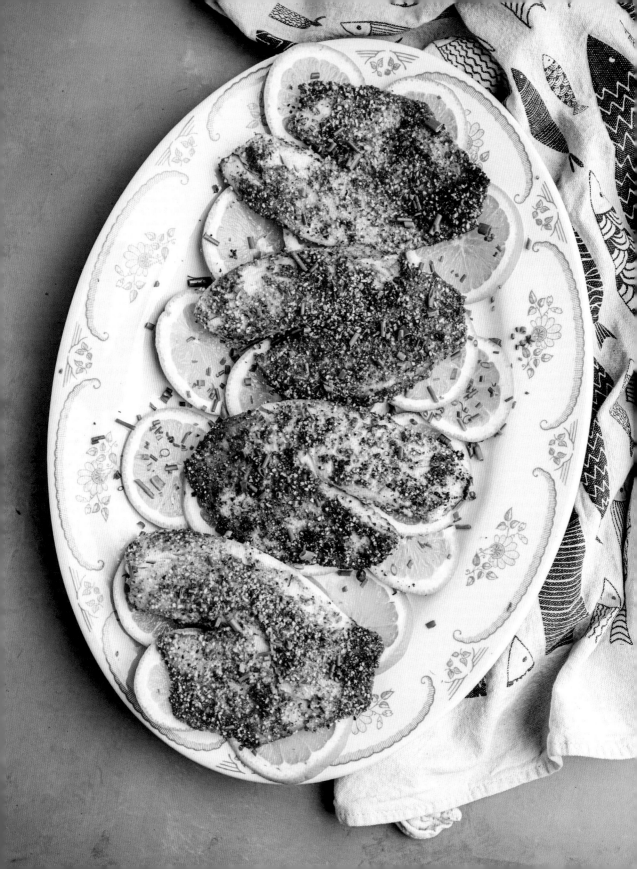

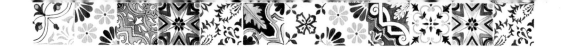

CRISPY ZA'ATAR TILAPIA
with Orange Slices

SERVES 4   Prep time: 10 minutes ✳ Cook time: 10 minutes

Writing a cookbook based on cognitive and mental health, we knew we had to pack it with super easy, yet super scrumptious seafood recipes—and this dish delivers. This tempting tilapia dish pairs sweet citrus with Mediterranean staples like za'atar and cumin, serving up several layers of flavor along with all the vital antioxidants, minerals, and omega-3s found in spices and fish. Serve these fillets with our Sautéed Greens with Honey-Tahini Sauce (page 90), Black Pepper and Coffee Roasted Carrots (page 81).

Using a Microplane or citrus zester, grate the zest from one orange into a shallow bowl or pie dish. Cut both oranges into thin rounds and arrange on a serving platter. Set aside.

Add the cornmeal, za'atar, salt, and pepper to the bowl with the orange zest and mix well. Dredge each piece of fish in the spice mixture until covered on each side.

In a large cast-iron skillet, heat the oil over medium-high heat. Carefully place each coated fillet into the hot oil and cook for 4 minutes. Flip the fillets and cook until the fish just starts to flake in the middle, 2 to 3 more minutes. Remove from the pan, place on top of the orange slices, sprinkle with chives, if desired and serve.

Healthy Kitchen Hack: Fresh or frozen, just about any type of fish fillet works great with this recipe. For other types of delicate white fish like flounder, grouper, or snapper, cooking times remain the same. For meatier fillets like salmon, tuna, or cod, add a few more minutes of cooking time per side or cook until a meat thermometer measures 145°F.

2 medium oranges

2 tablespoons cornmeal

2 teaspoons za'atar
(see Hack on page 115)

¼ teaspoon kosher
or sea salt

¼ teaspoon black pepper

4 (4-ounce) tilapia fillets
(skin-on or skinless)

2 tablespoons extra-virgin
olive oil

Chopped fresh chives,
for garnish (optional)

> 66
> *My husband and I really enjoyed this fish, from the oranges to the za'atar to the chives.*
>
> JOANNE FROM
> RADNOR, PA

PER SERVING: Calories: 220; Total Fat: 9g; Saturated Fat: 2g; Cholesterol: 58mg; Sodium: 182mg; Total Carbohydrates: 12g; Fiber: 2g; Protein: 24g

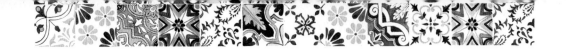

BROILED TROUT
with Coriander and Cilantro

SERVES 4   Prep time: 15 minutes   ✳   Cook time: 5 minutes

4 (4-ounce) fresh or thawed frozen skin-on trout fillets

½ teaspoon kosher or sea salt, divided

¼ teaspoon black pepper

1 lemon

⅔ cup plain whole-milk Greek yogurt or Homemade Yogurt (page 60)

2 tablespoons extra-virgin olive oil

1 teaspoon ground coriander (see Hack)

½ cup chopped fresh cilantro leaves and stems, plus more for garnish

Slathering fish in mayonnaise keeps it tender and juicy when cooking it under the high heat of the broiler—and, it turns out, that trick works just as well with our famously craveable "Mediterranean mayo," made with yogurt, olive oil, lemon, and salt. Besides using trout, Serena has made this speedy recipe dozens of times with different fish varieties, including Arctic char, salmon, and cod. Make it your go-to recipe to help your family eat two servings of seafood weekly for all the brain benefits.

Place the top oven rack about 4 inches below the broiler element. Preheat the broiler. Line a large rimmed baking sheet with aluminum foil and coat with cooking spray.

Place the trout skin side down on the lined baking sheet and sprinkle with ¼ teaspoon salt and the pepper. Tuck any thin ends under so the fillets are roughly the same thickness, then arrange the fillets down the center of the baking sheet so they will all be directly under the heat source.

Using a Microplane or citrus zester, grate the zest from the lemon into a medium bowl, then cut the lemon in half and squeeze in 2 tablespoons juice. Cut the remaining half into wedges and set aside for serving. Stir in the yogurt, oil coriander, and remaining ¼ teaspoon salt. Transfer half of this yogurt mixture to a small serving bowl and mix in the cilantro. Spread the remaining yogurt mixture over the tops and sides of each trout fillet.

Broil until the fish flakes easily and a few brown caramelized spots appear, 3 to 4 minutes.

Top the broiled fish with extra cilantro if desired, and serve it with the yogurt mixture on the side, along with the reserved lemon wedges for squeezing.

Healthy Kitchen Hack: This recipe uses three parts of the coriander plant: the leaves, stems, and seeds. (The fresh leaves of the plant are usually called cilantro in the US.) The stems are actually sweeter than the leaves, so always chop them to use in your recipe. If you've ever grown cilantro and it went to seed, those peppercorn-sized, round brown seeds can be dried and ground into dried coriander. Coriander seeds are commonly used in pickling spice mixes and in cuisines around the Mediterranean, especially in the Middle East and North Africa.

66

This easy recipe took less than 25 minutes. And I was very pleased with the outcome— the fillets were so moist and the sauce was delicious.

JACKIE FROM HOUSTON, TX

PER SERVING: Calories: 232; Total Fat: 13g; Saturated Fat: 3g; Cholesterol: 67mg; Sodium: 205mg; Total Carbohydrates: 3g; Fiber: 0g; Protein: 26g

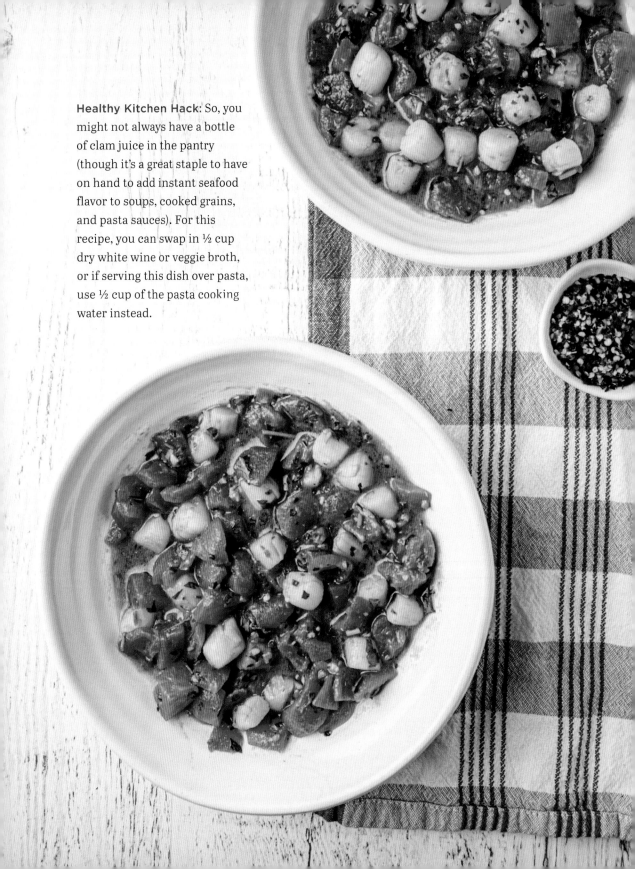

Healthy Kitchen Hack: So, you might not always have a bottle of clam juice in the pantry (though it's a great staple to have on hand to add instant seafood flavor to soups, cooked grains, and pasta sauces). For this recipe, you can swap in ½ cup dry white wine or veggie broth, or if serving this dish over pasta, use ½ cup of the pasta cooking water instead.

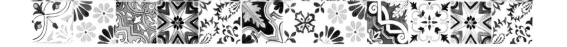

Scallops FRA DIAVOLO

SERVES 4 Prep time: 10 minutes ＊ Cook time: 25 minutes

Fra Diavolo ("Brother Devil"), the robust classic tomato sauce, is typically made with shrimp or lobster and served over linguine. In our version, we prepare it with quick-cooking bay scallops. Less expensive and more sustainable than sea scallops, these little mollusks deliver loads of flavor, which means fewer ingredients are needed to pull off a delectable dish. These tiny scallops also deliver big brain benefits through zinc, omega-3 fatty acids, and vitamin B12, which aid brain growth and memory retention. Enjoy them in this speedy, spicy sauce as is, over pasta, or with crusty bread slices to sop it all up.

3 tablespoons extra-virgin olive oil, divided

1 (1-pound) bag frozen bay scallops, thawed

6 garlic cloves, minced

¾–1 teaspoon crushed red pepper

½ cup clam juice (see Hack)

1 (28-ounce) can low-sodium diced tomatoes, undrained

½ cup chopped fresh parsley leaves and stems

Heat 2 tablespoons oil in a large skillet over medium heat. Add half of the scallops and cook, stirring gently and frequently, until milky white and firm, 3 to 4 minutes (depending on their size and package instructions). Using tongs or a slotted spoon, transfer the cooked scallops to a small bowl. Repeat with the remaining scallops.

Leaving the remaining scallop liquid in the skillet, return it to the stove over medium-low heat and add the remaining 1 tablespoon oil. Add the garlic and crushed red pepper and cook, stirring frequently, until fragrant, 2 minutes. Add the clam juice and, using a wooden spoon, scrape up the bottom of the skillet until the brown bits are incorporated into the liquid, about 1 minute.

Using a fine-mesh strainer or a slotted spoon, drain the juice from the bowl of scallops and add the juice to the skillet. Add the diced tomatoes with their juices, raise the heat to medium-high, and cook until the sauce just starts to simmer. Continue to simmer until it starts to reduce and thicken, 12 to 15 minutes. Stir in the scallops and heat for 1 to 2 minutes to rewarm. Remove from the heat, stir in the parsley, and serve.

PER SERVING: Calories: 292; Total Fat: 11g; Saturated Fat: 2g; Cholesterol: 40mg; Sodium: 515mg; Total Carbohydrates: 24g; Fiber: 4g; Protein: 26g

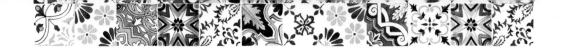

Clam and Leek
MINI POT PIES

SERVES 6 Prep time: 20 minutes ✳ Cook time: 50 minutes

2 tablespoons extra-virgin olive oil

2 leeks, trimmed and sliced

1 russet potato, scrubbed and cubed

1 carrot, scrubbed and diced

3 garlic cloves, minced

3 tablespoons all-purpose flour

1½ cups 2% milk

4 (6.5-ounce) cans minced or chopped clams, drained (liquid reserved; see Hack)

½ teaspoon dried thyme

¼ teaspoon black pepper

⅛ teaspoon cayenne pepper

1 large egg

1 refrigerated pie dough for 9-inch pie, room temperature

While pot pies may not seem all that Mediterranean, savory pastries featuring protein and vegetables likely originated in ancient Greece. This specific recipe isn't authentically Greek, but it does feature clams, a common shellfish varietal found in the Mediterranean Sea, paired with leeks, which are beloved by many countries in this region. Clams also are an excellent source of many nutrients critical to cognitive and mental health, including zinc, which can help improve memory. Enjoy the comfort—and nutrition!—of these cozy, individual ramekin meals.

Preheat the oven to 375°F. Place six (5-ounce) ramekins on a large rimmed baking sheet.

In a medium saucepan, heat the olive oil over medium heat. Add the leeks, potato, and carrot and cook, stirring occasionally, for 10 minutes, or until the vegetables start to soften. Add the garlic, and cook, stirring frequently, for 30 seconds. Stir in the flour and cook, stirring frequently, for 30 seconds. Whisk in the milk, ½ cup reserved clam juice, thyme, black pepper, and cayenne pepper and cook, whisking frequently, until the sauce starts to simmer and thicken, 2 to 3 minutes. Continue to whisk constantly as the sauce further thickens for about 1 minute. Remove the pot from the heat and mix in the clams. Ladle or pour the mixture evenly into the ramekins.

In a small bowl, whisk the egg with 1 tablespoon water, then brush the egg wash over the lip of each ramekin. Roll out the pie dough and cut into 6 equal pie wedges (triangles). Place a piece of dough over each ramekin, then shape it to cover the top. Crimp and seal to the lip. Brush more egg wash over the dough tops and make several slits on top of each. Place the sheet in the oven and bake for 30 to 35 minutes, until the crusts are golden brown. Let cool for 10 minutes before serving.

Healthy Kitchen Hack: Expand your horizons with these pot pies and swap in different seafood varieties like canned and drained tuna, salmon, or mackerel. Other options include raw shrimp (small or large cut in half) or firm raw fish like cod, salmon, or tilapia, cut into 1-inch pieces. You'll also need ½ cup bottled clam juice for this recipe; save the rest for a pasta sauce or soup recipe.

66

I enjoyed every bite! I could see myself ordering this at an oceanside restaurant by a fireplace with the cold winter winds blowing outside.

JOHN FROM HAVERTOWN, PA

PER SERVING: Calories: 409; Total Fat: 19g; Saturated Fat: 4g; Cholesterol: 174mg; Sodium: 792mg; Total Carbohydrates: 35g; Fiber: 4g; Protein: 26g

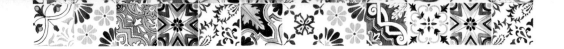

POTATO TORTILLA
with Mackerel and Peppers

SERVES 6 Prep time: 10 minutes ✳ Cook time: 20 minutes

1 (12-ounce) jar roasted red peppers, drained and chopped

7 large eggs

¼ cup chopped fresh parsley leaves and stems

2 tablespoons chopped fresh chives, divided

½ teaspoon smoked paprika

¼ teaspoon kosher or sea salt

¼ teaspoon black pepper

1 (4.4-ounce) can mackerel in olive oil, drained (oil reserved)

1 tablespoon extra-virgin olive oil

4½ cups frozen cubed potatoes or diced hash browns (from a 28- or 32-ounce package)

❝

Overall, this tortilla is really easy to make—it's filling and very enjoyable to eat!

KELLY FROM
MAYS LANDING, NJ

Taste the iconic flavors of sunny Spain in this classic potato tortilla, which is also referred to as a Spanish omelet. Typically served as a tapas or breakfast dish, here you can pair it with a salad and have it as a main course. But any time of day you enjoy it, you'll get a nice dose of choline from the eggs and omega-3s and vitamin D from the mackerel (or whichever canned fish you choose; see the Hack)—all vital nutrients for optimal brain function.

Put half of the chopped red peppers in a large bowl and set the remaining aside. Add the eggs, parsley, 1 tablespoon chives, smoked paprika, salt, and black pepper and whisk together. Add the mackerel, gently breaking the mackerel into small pieces with a fork and folding it into the egg mixture. Set aside.

Place the top oven rack about 6 inches below the broiler element. Preheat the broiler.

Pour the oil from the mackerel can and the 1 tablespoon olive oil into a 12-inch oven-safe skillet and heat over medium heat. Add the frozen potatoes to the pan and cook, stirring occasionally, to break apart any frozen clumps, until the potatoes are thawed and just starting to brown, about 10 minutes. Continue to cook the potatoes without stirring (so that they develop a bottom crust), for 4 more minutes. Pour in the egg mixture to cover the potatoes and stir occasionally until the eggs just start to set, about 3 minutes.

PER SERVING: Calories: 283; Total Fat: 11g; Saturated Fat: 3g; Cholesterol: 223mg; Sodium: 416mg; Total Carbohydrates: 35g; Fiber: 3g; Protein: 11g

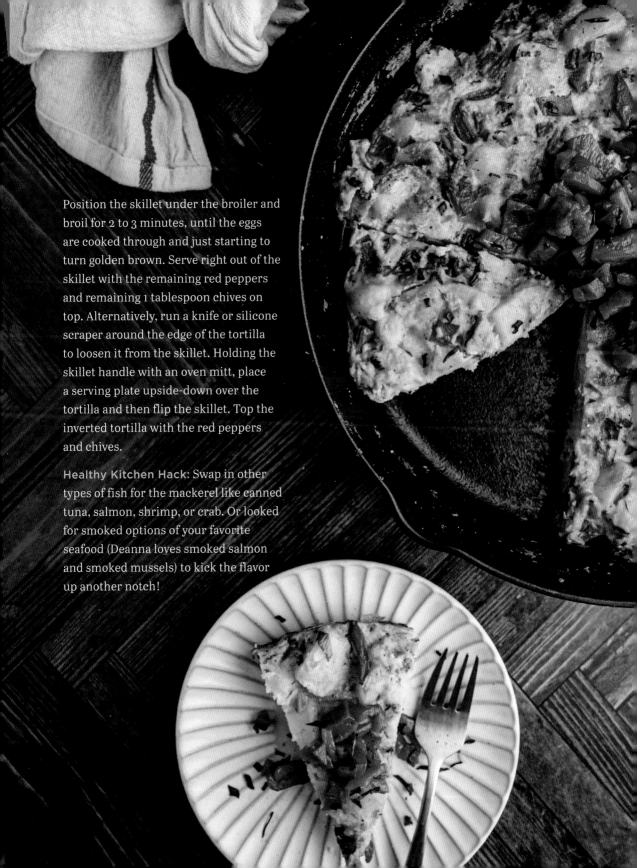

Position the skillet under the broiler and broil for 2 to 3 minutes, until the eggs are cooked through and just starting to turn golden brown. Serve right out of the skillet with the remaining red peppers and remaining 1 tablespoon chives on top. Alternatively, run a knife or silicone scraper around the edge of the tortilla to loosen it from the skillet. Holding the skillet handle with an oven mitt, place a serving plate upside-down over the tortilla and then flip the skillet. Top the inverted tortilla with the red peppers and chives.

Healthy Kitchen Hack: Swap in other types of fish for the mackerel like canned tuna, salmon, shrimp, or crab. Or looked for smoked options of your favorite seafood (Deanna loves smoked salmon and smoked mussels) to kick the flavor up another notch!

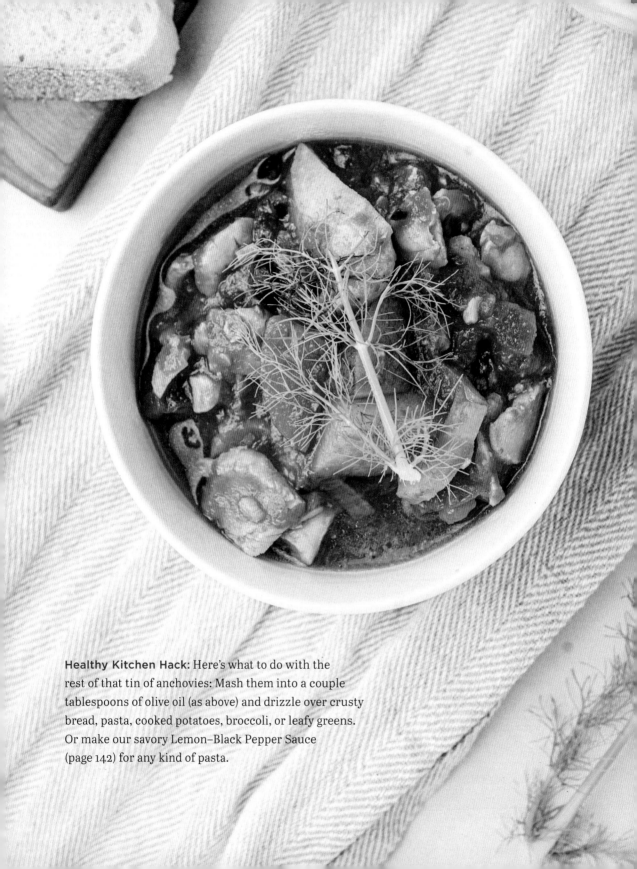

Healthy Kitchen Hack: Here's what to do with the rest of that tin of anchovies: Mash them into a couple tablespoons of olive oil (as above) and drizzle over crusty bread, pasta, cooked potatoes, broccoli, or leafy greens. Or make our savory Lemon–Black Pepper Sauce (page 142) for any kind of pasta.

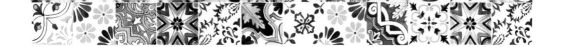

Puttanesca FISH STEW

SERVES 6 Prep time: 20 minutes ✳ Cook time: 30 minutes

Our twist on puttanesca—the classic garlic-olive-caper-tomato sauce for pasta—turns it into a robust seafood stew. We feature firm white fish and another fish that you might not even know is there: anchovies! As a staple ingredient in puttanesca, these little fishes melt into the olive oil and then disappear into the broth, adding a delectable savory layer (known as umami) that not even Serena's kids recognized as anchovies—and they're certainly not anchovy fans. Eating at least two servings of fish weekly is recommended for the long list of brain benefits that come from a variety of seafood. Serve with crusty bread to sop up all this succulent stew.

Heat 2 tablespoons oil in a large stockpot or Dutch oven over medium heat. Add the fennel and cook, stirring occasionally, until it begins to soften, 8 minutes. Push the fennel to the outer edges of the skillet. Add the remaining 1 tablespoon oil, anchovies, garlic, black pepper, and red pepper. Cook for 3 minutes, stirring frequently and mashing up the anchovies with a fork or a wooden spoon until they melt into the oil. Stir in the tomatoes, potatoes, olives, capers, thyme, and 2 cups water (use the water to rinse the tomato can). Increase the heat to high and bring to a boil. Reduce the heat to medium and cook until the potatoes are just soft when tested with a fork, about 8 minutes. Stir the fish into the stew. Cook until it just starts to flake with a fork, 4 to 6 minutes (depending on the thickness of the fish).

Serve from the pot topped with additional fennel fronds, if desired.

3 tablespoons extra-virgin olive oil, divided

1 cup thinly sliced fennel or celery, plus fennel fronds for garnish (optional)

3 anchovy fillets, drained and chopped, or 1½ teaspoons anchovy paste

4 garlic cloves, chopped

¼ teaspoon black pepper

¼ teaspoon crushed red pepper

1 (28-ounce) can low-sodium crushed tomatoes

6–8 small red or golden potatoes (about 1 pound), cut into ¾-inch pieces

½ cup chopped black olives

1 tablespoon capers, drained

2 teaspoons fresh thyme leaves or ¾ teaspoon dried thyme

1 pound fresh or thawed frozen cod or other firm white fish, cut into 1-inch pieces

PER SERVING: Calories: 257; Total Fat: 9g; Saturated Fat: 1g; Cholesterol: 37 mg; Sodium: 646 mg; Total Carbohydrates: 27g; Fiber: 5g; Protein: 18g

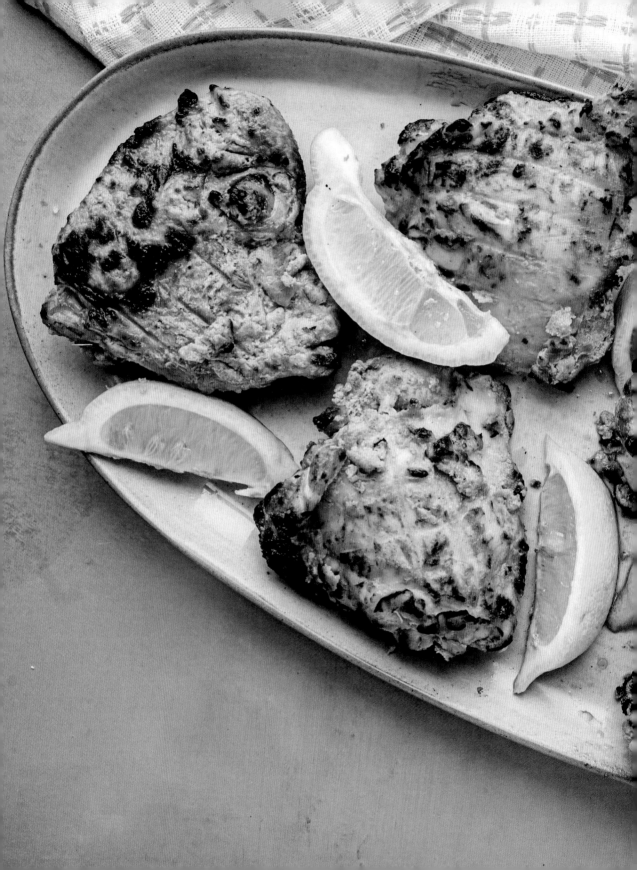

MEAT & POULTRY

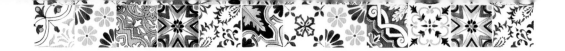

STEAK AU POIVRE
with Herbes de Provence Potato Wedges

SERVES 4   Prep time: 40 minutes   ✳   Cook time: 35 minutes

1 pound boneless beef
round sirloin tip steak
or top round steak
(about ¾ inch thick)

½ teaspoon kosher
or sea salt, divided

1½ pounds large russet
potatoes, scrubbed
and cut lengthwise into
½-inch-wide wedges

2 tablespoons extra-virgin
olive oil, divided

1 teaspoon
herbes de Provence
(see Hack on page 119)

1 tablespoon whole
black peppercorns or
1½ teaspoons coarsely
ground black pepper

½ cup torn fresh
basil leaves

Steak au poivre is the classic French dish in which steak is encrusted with fresh ground black pepper, pan seared, and served with a cream-based pan sauce. Our brain-friendly, freshened-up approach skips the sauce in favor of topping the rich meat with tender green basil, and we oven-roast the steak at a low temperature to heat it gently, keep it tender, and allow some of the saturated fat to drip away. After slightly cooling, cutting the steak against the grain is another tenderizing trick. And those black peppercorns are gold-star spices for antioxidant power; grinding fresh yourself (instead of pre-ground black pepper) keeps even more antioxidants intact.

Place the steak on a plate and sprinkle all over with ¼ teaspoon salt. Set aside at room temperature for at least 30 minutes to allow the steak to absorb the salt for better flavor.

Arrange the oven racks in the upper-middle and lower-middle positions. Preheat the oven to 400°F. Coat two large rimmed baking sheets with cooking spray. Place a wire rack on one of the sheets and coat with cooking spray.

In a large bowl, toss the potatoes with 1 tablespoon oil, the herbes de Provence, and the remaining ¼ teaspoon salt. Spread out the potatoes on the empty prepared baking sheet. Place on the lower oven rack and roast for 15 minutes.

Meanwhile, if using whole peppercorns, place them in a zip-top plastic bag and crush with a rolling pin or heavy skillet until cracked into coarsely ground pieces. (Or crush using a pepper grinder.) Firmly press the cracked peppercorn into both sides of the steak, then place it on the wire rack on the other baking sheet.

Reduce the oven temperature to 300°F and remove the potatoes to stir, then place them back on the lower oven rack (there's no need to wait for the oven to come down to 300°F). Place the baking sheet with the steak on the upper oven rack. Roast both for 15 to 17 minutes, until the potatoes are just fork-tender and the internal temperature of the steak is 100°F when measured with a meat thermometer.

When the steak and potatoes are about 5 minutes from being done, heat a large cast-iron skillet on the stovetop over medium-high heat for 5 minutes. Pour in the remaining 1 tablespoon oil to heat. Remove both baking sheets from the oven; set the potatoes aside. Using tongs, carefully transfer the steak to the hot oil in the skillet. Sear the steak until it develops a brown crust, about 1 minute. Flip the steak (being careful to avoid dislodging the peppercorns) and cook until the other side develops a brown crust and the internal temperature reaches the butcher-recommended medium-rare doneness of 120°F to 130°F on a meat thermometer, 1 to 2 minutes (or, if you prefer, about another 2 minutes to reach 135°F to 140°F for medium).

Transfer the steak to a cutting board and cover loosely with aluminum foil; let rest for 5 minutes. Cut into thin strips and sprinkle with the basil. Serve with the potato wedges.

Healthy Kitchen Hack: Fresh herbs on bold, salty, umami meat is a great way to balance and perk up the savory flavors. Try our Green Olive Salsa Verde (page 89) or our Speedy Pesto Sauce (page 130) in place of the basil with this steak or use them on top of other simple grilled or broiled proteins like chicken or fish.

> *The basil on top of the steak was really nice! And the flavor of the steak with the cracked peppercorns was so good. My family hadn't tried herbes de Provence before, and we liked that, too.*
>
> CHRIS FROM MORRISVILLE, NC

PER SERVING: Calories: 343; Total Fat: 11g; Saturated Fat: 3g; Cholesterol: 67mg; Sodium: 228mg; Total Carbohydrates: 32g; Fiber: 3g; Protein: 29g

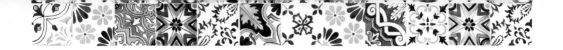

LEBANESE SPICED CABBAGE ROLLS *with Rice*

SERVES 4   Prep time: 20 minutes   ✳   Cook time: 45 minutes

1 tablespoon plus
1 teaspoon extra-virgin
olive oil, divided

1 small cabbage
(about 4 inches
in diameter)

1 small onion, chopped

½ teaspoon
ground cinnamon

½ teaspoon cumin seeds
or ground cumin

½ teaspoon kosher
or sea salt

¼ teaspoon black pepper

1 pound ground beef
(80–90% lean)

1½ cups cooked brown rice

¼ cup tomato paste

2 tablespoons raisins

¼ cup finely chopped
fresh mint, parsley, or
cilantro leaves and stems

1 lemon, cut into wedges
(optional)

The Lebanese flavor combo of cinnamon, cumin, and mint makes these stuffed meat pockets memorable (pun intended!). If you can roll a wrap, you can roll this savory filling up into something new for dinner tonight. Plus we share a surprising trick for making cabbage leaves pliable and easy to peel off the cabbage head. Cabbage is a cruciferous vegetable brimming with fiber and brain-friendly antioxidants, along with other nutrients to help keep blood flowing smoothly to the brain.

Preheat the oven to 375°F. Brush a Dutch oven or 2-quart casserole dish with 1 teaspoon oil.

In a large stockpot or Dutch oven, bring about 3 inches of water to a boil. Using a kitchen spider or two large spoons, lower the head of cabbage into the water and cover the pot. Boil for about 3 minutes, until the leaves are pliable and tender-crisp. Carefully remove the head and cool slightly. The leaves will separate easily as you gently peel off eight leaves. (Save the remaining cabbage for another use.)

Heat the remaining 1 tablespoon oil in a large skillet over medium heat. Add the onion and cook, stirring occasionally, until it starts to soften, 5 minutes. Add the cinnamon, cumin, salt, and pepper and cook, stirring frequently, for 1 minute. Add the ground beef and cook, breaking up the chunks with a wooden spoon and stirring occasionally, until the beef is cooked through and no longer pink, about 8 minutes. Stir in the rice, tomato paste, and raisins and cook, stirring, until the tomato paste is well incorporated, 2 to 3 minutes. Remove from the heat and cool slightly.

continued on page 208

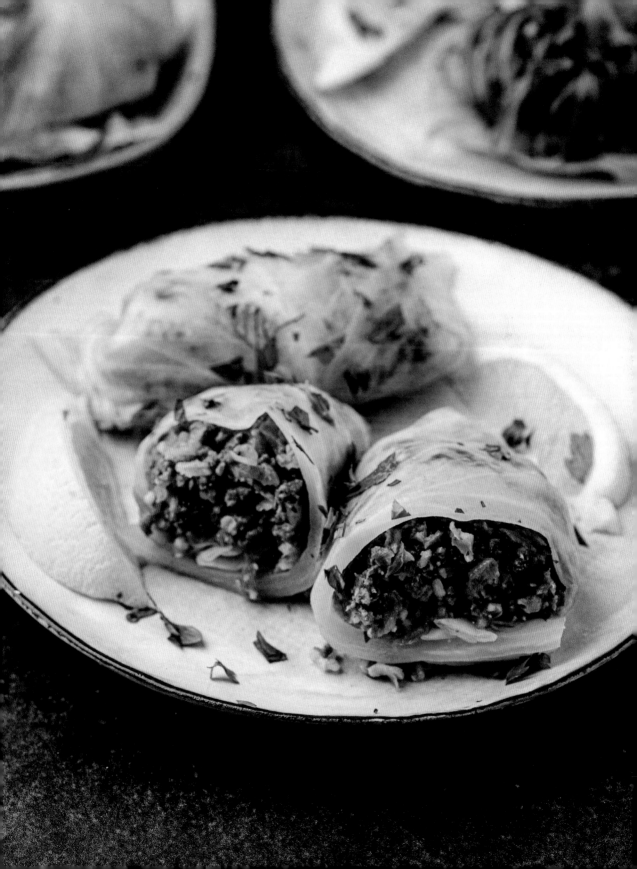

continued from page 206

Spoon ⅓ cup of the meat stuffing onto the end of a cabbage leaf (not the core end). Roll into a wrap, rolling in the direction the leaf naturally curves and folding in the edges while rolling. Place on a plate seam side down. Repeat with the remaining cabbage leaves and meat (there will be leftover meat stuffing). Spoon the leftover stuffing into the Dutch oven and spread out to cover the bottom of the pot. Gently place the cabbage rolls on top of the stuffing, still seam side down, and pour ½ cup water over the rolls. Cover with a lid or aluminum foil and bake for 25 minutes, or until heated through.

When ready to serve, uncover and sprinkle with the fresh herbs. Serve with lemon wedges for squeezing, if desired.

Healthy Kitchen Hack: Rolling up these cabbage rolls is easy, but if you don't have time to bake them, try one of these two shortcuts: (1) Roll up the cabbage and filling as directed and then serve immediately at room temperature, or refrigerate for later to serve cold as is customary in some Lebanese families. (2) Skip the cabbage boiling step and instead, add about 3 cups shredded cabbage with the onion to the oil in the skillet and cook until tender-crisp. Follow the remaining instructions to add the spices and then the meat. Serve as a skillet dinner of deconstructed cabbage rolls.

PER SERVING: Calories: 351; Total Fat: 14g; Saturated Fat: 4g; Cholesterol: 71mg; Sodium: 256mg; Total Carbohydrates: 31g; Fiber: 4g; Protein: 27g

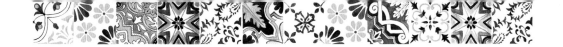

Honey-Tahini
PORK TENDERLOIN

SERVES 4 Prep time: 30 minutes ✳ Cook time: 20 minutes

These juicy pork tenderloins are rolled in a sweet and nutty glaze made with an ingredient you may have had only in hummus: tahini, or sesame seed butter. This Middle Eastern staple ingredient helps the honey and sesame seeds stick to the tenderloin while sealing in the juices to keep the meat succulent. Sesame seeds (both the whole seeds and the seeds in tahini) contain potent antioxidants and other nutrients to help guard against dementia. And the honey contains oligosaccharides, a specific sugar that serves as prebiotic food for a healthy gut—and a healthy gut can mean a healthy brain. Whip up this easy protein-packed meal on any weekday with just a few ingredients.

2 (10- to 12-ounce) pork tenderloins

½ teaspoon kosher or sea salt

¼ teaspoon black pepper

¼ cup honey

¼ cup tahini

2 tablespoons sesame seeds, divided

4 scallions (green onions), green and white parts, thinly sliced

1 tablespoon lemon juice

Preheat the oven to 450°F. Line a large rimmed baking sheet with aluminum foil and coat well with cooking spray.

Place both pork pieces on the foil-lined sheet and sprinkle evenly with the salt and pepper. Let sit at room temperature for 10 to 20 minutes.

In a medium bowl, whisk together the honey, tahini, and 1 tablespoon hot water until smooth. Pour the honey mixture onto a shallow plate. Put 1 tablespoon sesame seeds on another plate. Roll one pork tenderloin in the honey mixture to coat evenly, then roll in the sesame seeds and place back on the foil. Add the remaining 1 tablespoon sesame seeds to the plate and repeat the coating process with the remaining tenderloin. Reserve the extra glaze on the plate to make the honey-tahini sauce for serving; see the Hack.

continued on page 210

continued from page 209

Roast for 18 to 22 minutes, until the internal temperature of the pork reaches 140°F on a meat thermometer. Transfer the pork to a cutting board and let it rest for 5 to 10 minutes.

To make the sauce, while the meat roasts, scrape the remaining glaze off the plate and into a liquid measuring cup. Add 1 tablespoon lemon juice and enough water to make ½ cup total liquid. Cook in a small pot over medium heat until boiling, stirring frequently. Boil for 1 minute. (As the sauce warms, it will first separate and curdle, but will then turn into a smooth cohesive sauce.)

To serve, spoon the sauce over the pork slices. Slice, sprinkle with the scallions, and serve with the honey-tahini sauce.

Healthy Kitchen Hack: This recipe's sauce-making technique can be used with leftover marinades in many other recipes, too. Make it a habit to use up your marinades by boiling for 1 minute and get the most out of your ingredients!

PER SERVING: (including optional sauce): Calories: 246; Total Fat: 9g; Saturated Fat: 2g; Cholesterol: 74mg; Sodium: 226mg; Total Carbohydrates: 15g; Fiber: 1g; Protein: 26g

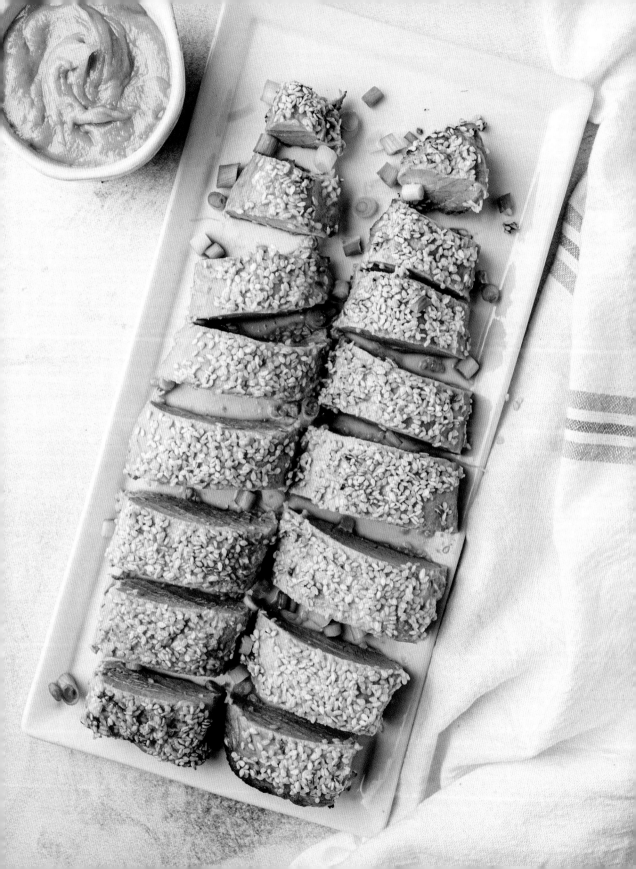

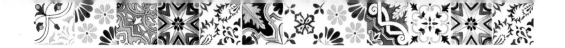

PALESTINIAN KAFTA
with Lots of Parsley

SERVES 6 Prep time: 45 minutes ✳ Cook time: 20 minutes

1 cup bulgur

1½ cups chopped fresh parsley leaves and stems (about 1 bunch)

1 medium onion, very finely chopped (see Hack)

1 teaspoon ground cinnamon

½ teaspoon kosher or sea salt

½ teaspoon black pepper

¼ teaspoon ground allspice

1 pound ground lamb

1 large egg, lightly beaten

1 recipe Creamy Cucumber Salad with Sesame Dressing, for serving (page 66; optional)

Kafta or kofta are a family of meatball and meatloaf dishes common in the Middle East, the Balkans, and South and Central Asia. The inspiration for this comforting meatloaf-like kafta comes from Serena's friend Nabil, and the recipe includes, at his insistence, "lots" of parsley. It's how he learned to make it from his mother, growing up in his family's Palestinian home, just two blocks from the Mediterranean Sea. Parsley is good for the brain and really good in this recipe, so there's a whole bunch, literally (they do say moms know best).

Preheat the oven to 400°F. Coat a 9 × 13-inch baking pan with cooking spray.

In a large bowl, stir together the bulgur and 2 cups boiling water. Cover the bowl with a plate and set aside for 15 minutes, or until the bulgur is soft. Drain the excess water and let cool for at least 10 minutes, stirring occasionally.

To the bulgur, add the parsley, onion, cinnamon, salt, pepper, and allspice and mix well. Add the lamb and egg and mix with your hands until well combined.

Using your hands, spread the mixture into the prepared pan and flatten until smooth. Using a butter knife, score the meat mixture into 18 equal squarish portions, separating each portion so you can see a little of the pan. Bake for 18 to 22 minutes, until the internal temperature of the lamb measures 160°F on a meat thermometer.

Cut the kafta into portions along the scored lines and serve straight from the pan or transfer the portions to a serving platter. Serve with the cucumber salad, if desired.

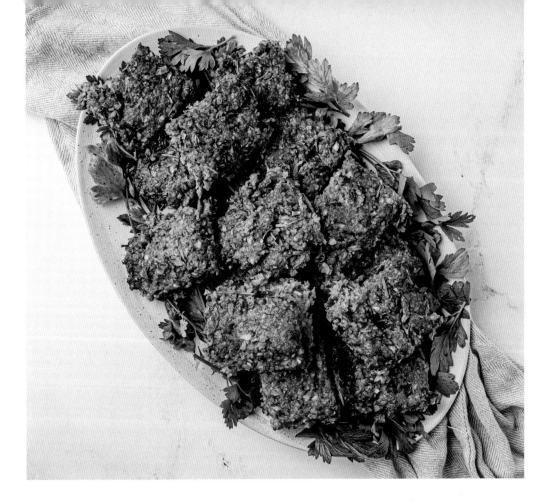

Healthy Kitchen Hack: The onion should be very finely chopped for this recipe. Make sure your kitchen knife is sharp or break out a mini food processor for the task. Or, you can make the whole recipe in a regular-size food processor. Use it to chop the parsley and onion, then add the spices and bulgur and pulse to combine. Add the meat and pulse a few times until combined. In our other books, we've taught to not overmix ground meat as it results in smashed-together burgers/meatballs that seem less tender and appealing. But thanks to the moisture of the bulgur along with fat-rich lamb, this pressed "meatloaf"—even when combined in a processor—still results in a juicy kafta.

> ❝
> *Even though I have never, ever added "burgul" (as we call bulgur) to my kafta, I approve of this recipe from my friend Serena. It also has enough parsley, but just barely!*
>
> NABIL FROM
> SIOUX FALLS, SD

PER SERVING: Calories: 309; Total Fat: 18g; Saturated Fat: 8g; Cholesterol: 55mg; Sodium: 252mg; Total Carbohydrates: 21g; Fiber: 4g; Protein: 16g

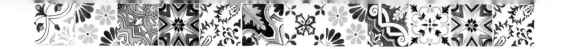

CHICKEN KEBABS
with Grapes and Olives

SERVES 4 Prep time: 30 minutes ❊ Cook time: 10 minutes

1 lemon

2 tablespoon extra-virgin olive oil

1 tablespoon minced fresh rosemary

⅛ teaspoon kosher or sea salt

⅛ teaspoon black pepper

8 ounces purple or green seedless grapes (about 48)

1 (6-ounce) can pitted green or black olives, drained

1 pound skinless, boneless chicken thighs, cut into 1-inch pieces

Ever thought of pairing grapes with olives? These two fruits (yes, olives are a fruit!) are a perfect Mediterranean combo thanks to their appearance, complementary sweet and buttery flavors, and, of course, brain-boosting nutrients. Both contain unique polyphenols that assist with healthy blood flow to the brain. So, both your brain and your taste buds are in for a treat the next time you grill and serve up these seriously scrumptious chicken kebabs!

Using a Microplane or citrus zester, grate the zest from the lemon into a large bowl, then cut the lemon in half and squeeze in the juice from one half. Cut the remaining half into wedges and set aside for serving. To the bowl of lemon zest and juice, add the oil, the rosemary, salt, and pepper and whisk to combine. Add the grapes and olives and carefully toss to coat. Using a slotted spoon, transfer the olives and grapes to a small bowl and set aside.

Add the chicken to the large bowl with the remaining lemon mixture and toss to coat. Cover with a plate and marinate at room temperature for 15 to 20 minutes. (If making ahead, cover and chill all the ingredients for up to 12 hours in the refrigerator. Set out at room temperature for 20 minutes before grilling.)

Thread the chicken onto twelve (10- to 12-inch) metal or wooden skewers, keeping the chunks close together so the meat stays juicy. Then thread the grapes and olives onto the same skewers.

PER SERVING: (3 skewers): Calories: 280; Total Fat: 15g; Saturated Fat: 3g; Cholesterol: 107mg; Sodium: 408mg; Total Carbohydrates: 14g; Fiber: 2g; Protein: 23g

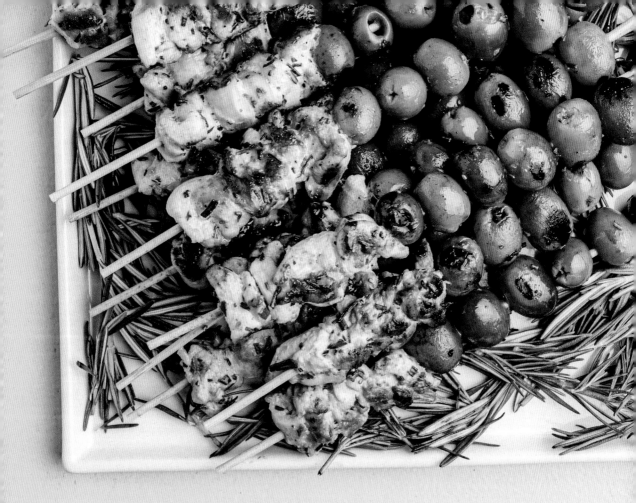

Coat the cold cooking grate of an outdoor grill with cooking spray, then preheat the grill to 400°F (or heat a stovetop grill pan to medium-high heat). Place the skewers on the grill and cook, turning every 2 to 3 minutes, until the chicken is cooked through and just barely charred, 8 to 10 minutes total. Remove the skewers from the grill and let rest for at least 5 minutes to allow the juices to set, then serve with the reserved lemon wedges for squeezing.

Healthy Kitchen Hack: Got extra fresh grapes? Here are two ways to make them special: (1) Place grapes on a parchment-lined rimmed baking sheet and freeze until firm, then store in an airtight container in the freezer for a mini ice-pop snack. (2) Scatter olive oil–drizzled grapes on a parchment-lined rimmed baking sheet and roast at 400°F for about 20 minutes. Sprinkle with salt and use to top yogurt, ice cream, or salads.

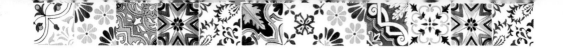

Pan-Fried
PARMESAN-PECAN CHICKEN

SERVES 6 Prep time: 15 minutes ✳ Cook time: 20 minutes

6 (4-ounce) boneless, skinless chicken breasts, cut into 6 pieces

⅔ cup pecans, finely chopped (see Hack)

⅓ cup cornmeal

3 tablespoons grated Parmesan cheese

½ teaspoon dried thyme

½ teaspoon cayenne pepper

¼ teaspoon kosher or sea salt

¼ teaspoon black pepper

½ cup plain 2% Greek yogurt or Homemade Yogurt (page 60)

1 tablespoon Dijon mustard

2 tablespoons extra-virgin olive oil, divided

Bring on the nutty, the cheesy, and the spicy heat! This chicken dish features classic Mediterranean ingredients combined into an irresistible crunchy coating, while delivering some important nutrients for mood balance and cognitive well-being (gotta love those nuts and spices). Serve it with our Berry Smart Seeded Dressing over Greens (page 64) or our Creamy Cucumber Salad with Sesame Dressing (page 66) to balance the slow burn and bolster your daily "pro-brain" nutrient intake.

Place one chicken breast between two pieces of parchment paper. Using the smooth side of a meat mallet, metal ladle, or small pan, pound the breast to an even ¾-inch thickness. Repeat with the same parchment with the remaining breasts. Set aside.

Put the pecans, cornmeal, Parmesan, thyme, cayenne pepper, salt, and black pepper in a shallow bowl and mix well. In a separate shallow bowl, whisk together the yogurt, mustard, and ¼ cup water.

Dip one piece of chicken in the yogurt mixture, coating both sides. Let any excess yogurt drip back into the bowl. Dredge the yogurt-coated chicken in the pecan mixture, fully coating both sides. Place the coated piece of chicken on a plate, then repeat the process with the remaining pieces.

Heat 1 tablespoon oil in a large cast-iron skillet over medium heat. When the oil is hot, carefully add 3 chicken pieces and cook, flipping halfway through, until a meat thermometer registers 165°F, 8 to 10 minutes total. Transfer the chicken to a serving plate. Wipe the skillet clean and add the remaining 1 tablespoon oil. Once heated, repeat the cooking process with the remaining chicken pieces. Serve immediately.

Healthy Kitchen Hack: When a recipe calls for finely chopped nuts, put down the knife and use your mini food processor or high-powered blender instead. A couple of pulses or seconds will do the trick for a crumb-like texture. You can use it to make your own nut meal, flour, or butter, too: A few more pulses will turn those finely chopped nuts into a nut meal or a flour. And if you keep the processor or blender running, you'll end up with a nut paste, which you can turn into nut butter by continuing the "blend" for several minutes, stopping from time to time to scrape down the bowl. The natural oils released from the nuts turn it into a smooth and creamy butter.

66
I liked the crunchy coating of the cornmeal and nuts. My husband loved this recipe and said, "Don't change a thing!"

REBECCA FROM
ESCONDIDO, CA

PER SERVING: Calories: 314; Total Fat: 18g; Saturated Fat: 3g; Cholesterol: 87mg; Sodium: 278mg; Total Carbohydrates: 8g; Fiber: 2g; Protein: 30g

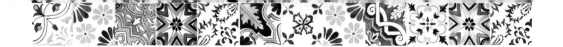

North African
SPICED YOGURT CHICKEN

SERVES 6 Prep time: 40 minutes ✳ Cook time: 15 minutes

6 (6-ounce) bone-in chicken thighs, skin removed and fat trimmed

2 lemons

1 tablespoon extra-virgin olive oil

½ teaspoon kosher or sea salt

1¼ teaspoons ground turmeric

1 teaspoon garlic powder

1 teaspoon smoked paprika

1 teaspoon ground cumin

½ teaspoon black pepper

1 (2-inch) piece ginger

⅔ cup plain whole-milk Greek yogurt or Homemade Yogurt (page 60)

¼ cup chopped fresh mint leaves and stems (optional)

This chicken thigh recipe is inspired by the popular North African spice blend ras el hanout (meaning "top shelf"), which can include up to 50 spices, including brain-benefitting ground cumin, black pepper, ginger, and turmeric. And the yogurt makes for a magical marinade, guaranteeing moist and perfectly spiced chicken every time.

Make 2 slashes (about ¼ inch deep) in the fleshy side of each chicken thigh; set aside.

Using a Microplane or citrus zester, grate the zest from one lemon into a large bowl, then cut the lemon in half and squeeze in the juice. Whisk in the oil, salt, turmeric, garlic powder, paprika, cumin, and pepper. Add the chicken and toss to coat. Cover the bowl with a plate and let the chicken marinate at room temperature for 20 minutes.

Place the top oven rack about 6 inches below the broiler element. Preheat the broiler. Line a large rimmed baking sheet with aluminum foil and place a wire cooling rack on top; coat the rack with cooking spray.

Remove the ginger peel with a vegetable peeler or scrape off with a spoon. Using a Microplane or the small holes on the box grater, grate the ginger until you have about 1 tablespoon. Put the ginger in a small bowl, add the yogurt, and whisk to combine.

When the chicken has finished marinating, add the ginger-yogurt mixture to the bowl and, using a fork or tongs, toss with the chicken to coat.

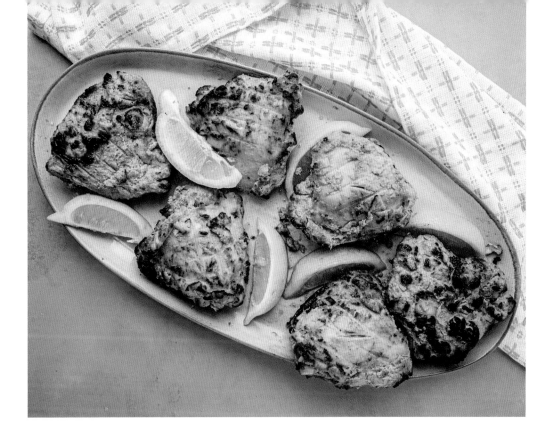

Pick up each chicken thigh over the bowl, let the excess yogurt mixture drip off, and then place the chicken, cut side down, on the prepared rack on the baking sheet. Broil for 8 to 12 minutes, flipping halfway through, until lightly charred on both sides and a meat thermometer inserted into the meaty part reads 165°F. (Turn the chicken a third time during cooking if you like a lighter char versus a darker char.)

Cut the remaining lemon into wedges. Serve the chicken topped with the mint, if desired, along with the lemon wedges for squeezing.

Healthy Kitchen Hack: As a savory ingredient, yogurt acts as a protective blanket around meat and poultry as it cooks. But a yogurt (or any acid) marinade can make meat mushy if it sits too long, so limit the marinating time to 1 hour at most.

66

I raved about this to my friends. It's easy to make and is packed with protein, which I recommend to my sports nutrition clients.

KEVIN FROM
SAN LUIS OBISPO, CA

PER SERVING: Calories: 242; Total Fat: 10g; Saturated Fat: 3g; Cholesterol: 144mg; Sodium: 314mg; Total Carbohydrates: 4g; Fiber: 1g; Protein: 33g

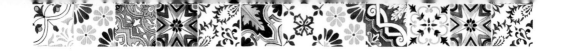

BRAISED CHICKEN KAPAMA
over Orzo

SERVES 6   Prep time: 10 minutes   ✳ Cook time: 40 minutes

2 tablespoons extra-virgin olive oil, divided

1½ pounds boneless, skinless chicken thighs

1 teaspoon ground cinnamon, divided

¼ teaspoon kosher or sea salt

1 onion, diced

1 carrot, scrubbed and shredded

½ teaspoon black pepper

¼ cup dry red wine or 1 tablespoon red wine vinegar plus 3 tablespoons water

1 (28-ounce) can low-sodium crushed tomatoes

2 teaspoons dried oregano

8 ounces orzo

¼ cup grated Parmesan cheese

Chicken kapama is classic Greek comfort food with many variations, but the common thread is the tomato sauce spiced with warm cinnamon (which is also featured in our Spiced Tomato Soup with Fried Halloumi, page 96, and our Mushroom Pastitsio "Baked" Pasta, page 148). The intoxicating scent of cinnamon cooking can be pleasing or even relaxing to your mind and mood. As it stews, this dish may draw people into the kitchen, which can become a comforting part of your family dinner routine, especially on those colder, blustery days.

Heat 1 tablespoon oil in a large pot or Dutch oven over medium heat. Rub the chicken thighs with ¼ teaspoon cinnamon and the salt and then add them to the pot. Cook for 5 minutes, flip, and cook for 5 more minutes (they will not be cooked through). Transfer the chicken to a plate and set aside.

Add the remaining 1 tablespoon oil to the pot. Add the onion, carrot, and pepper and cook, first scraping the bottom for the chicken bits and then stirring occasionally, for about 5 minutes, until the vegetables soften. Add the remaining ¾ teaspoon cinnamon and red wine and cook, stirring occasionally, until the liquid evaporates, about 1 minute. Add the tomatoes, oregano, and 1¼ cups water (from rinsing out the tomato can) and cook, stirring occasionally, until the sauce starts to simmer, about 5 minutes. Reduce the heat to medium-low and return the chicken to the pot, along with any accumulated juices on the plate. Cover and cook for at least 15 minutes for the flavors to meld and the chicken to reach 165°F on a meat thermometer.

While the chicken cooks, cook the orzo according to the package instructions. Drain, then transfer to a serving platter and mix in the Parmesan cheese.

Top the orzo with the chicken pieces and sauce and serve.

Healthy Kitchen Hack: In a chicken rut? Make a meat kapama: Swap in beef shoulder or beef chuck roast and cook for at least 1 hour, adding more liquid as needed. Or make it vegetarian: skip the chicken and mix in 2 (15-ounce) cans of chickpeas, kidney beans, or white beans with their liquid at the step above where you would return the chicken to the pot.

66

My boys loved this—even with the cinnamon—and asked for seconds!

CLAIRE FROM HAVERTOWN, PA

PER SERVING: Calories: 395; Total Fat: 12g; Saturated Fat: 3g; Cholesterol: 110mg; Sodium: 521mg; Total Carbohydrates: 42g; Fiber: 5g; Protein: 31g

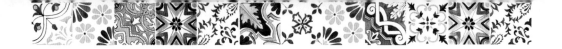

Blueberry
TURKEY PANZANELLA

SERVES 6 Prep time: 20 minutes

2 cups chopped cooked turkey breast (1-inch pieces)

2 cups cubed stale or toasted baguette or other crusty bread (1-inch pieces)

2 cups fresh blueberries, divided (see Hack)

1 cup grape tomatoes, halved

½ cup diced red onion

⅓ cup crumbled Gorgonzola cheese

⅓ cup chopped pecans

1 lemon

¼ cup extra-virgin olive oil

2 teaspoons honey

¼ teaspoon kosher or sea salt

¼ teaspoon black pepper

1 cup fresh mint leaves and stems, torn

If you've read our other cookbooks, you know Deanna loves to make panzanella. The traditional Italian tomato and bread peasant salad is an ideal base recipe to use up leftovers—and this turkey version was first created after one Thanksgiving. But the star of this dinner salad is the blueberry, a superhero food when it comes to brain health research, where powerful berry antioxidants have shown to help improve attention, memory, and even mood. So, it's really a no-brainer (pardon the pun) to get this panzanella into your meal rotation.

In a large salad bowl, toss together the turkey, bread, 1½ cups blueberries, tomatoes, onion, Gorgonzola, and pecans.

Right before serving, using a Microplane or citrus zester, grate the zest from the lemon into a blender, then cut the lemon in half and squeeze in the juice. Add the remaining ½ cup blueberries, oil, honey, salt, and pepper and blend until the blueberries are pulverized.

Drizzle the dressing over the panzanella and gently toss. Add the mint, gently toss again, and serve.

Tip: If the dressing sits for a bit before you use it, it can seize up. Simply run it again in the blender or whisk in a tablespoon of water to thin it out.

Healthy Kitchen Hack: Not blueberry season? No problem! Swap in frozen blueberries or any frozen berry you'd like. After thawing, drain the berries and use the juice to thin out the dressing as needed.

PER SERVING: Calories: 385; Total Fat: 18g; Saturated Fat: 4g; Cholesterol: 66mg; Sodium: 357mg; Total Carbohydrates: 30g; Fiber: 5g; Protein: 29g

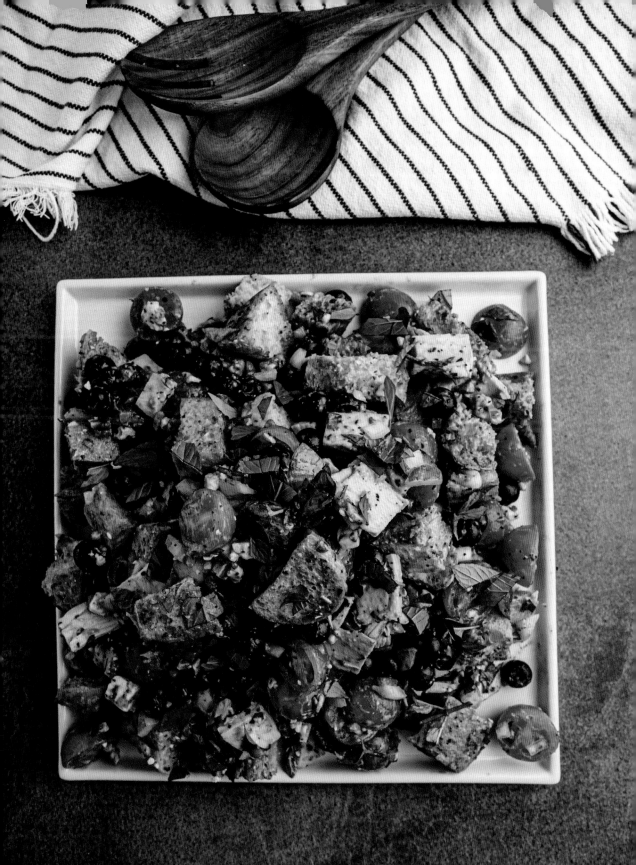

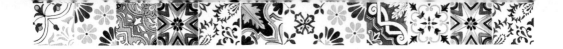

POMEGRANATE CHICKEN
with Turmeric Pistachio Rice

SERVES 6   Prep time: 15 minutes   ✳   Cook time: 45 minutes

1 lemon

½ cup pomegranate juice

3 tablespoons extra-virgin olive oil, divided

2 tablespoons honey

2 garlic cloves, minced

1 teaspoon kosher or sea salt, divided

½ teaspoon black pepper, divided

1½ pounds boneless, skinless chicken breasts

1 onion, chopped and divided

1¼ cups brown or wild rice

1 teaspoon ground turmeric

½ teaspoon ground cumin

½ cup shelled pistachios

¾ cup chopped fresh cilantro leaves and stems

Throughout the Mediterranean, chicken is often paired with fresh fruit, dried fruit, and/or fruit juice for succulent results. Here antioxidant-powered pomegranate juice mixed with honey and aromatics becomes a jewel-colored marinade and cooking sauce for chicken breasts. We serve it with whole-grain brown rice spiced with golden yellow turmeric and gorgeous green pistachios that give a crunch—vibrantly colored ingredients packed with nutrients to protect your brain and lighten your mood.

Preheat the oven to 450°F. Coat a 9-inch square baking pan with cooking spray.

Using a Microplane or citrus zester, grate the zest from the lemon into a large bowl, then cut the lemon in half and squeeze in the juice from half of the lemon (save the remaining lemon half for another use). Add the pomegranate juice, 2 tablespoons oil, the honey, garlic, ¼ teaspoon salt, and ¼ teaspoon pepper and whisk. Add the chicken and half of the onion and mix until everything is coated. Pour into the prepared baking pan and set aside to marinate at room temperature (or refrigerate for up to 1 hour) while you prep the rice.

In a medium pot, heat the remaining 1 tablespoon oil over medium heat. Add the remaining onion and cook, stirring occasionally, for 5 minutes. Add the rice, turmeric, and cumin and cook, stirring frequently, for 1 minute. Stir in the amount of water called for on the package instructions for 1¼ cups of rice, along with the remaining ¾ teaspoon salt.

Bring to a boil, cover, and lower the heat to medium-low. Cook according to the time on the package instructions or until the rice is cooked through and the liquid is absorbed. Remove the pot from the heat.

While the rice cooks, put the chicken in the oven and bake for 22 to 25 minutes, until a meat thermometer inserted into the thick part of the breast registers 165F° and the liquid has reduced a bit.

Stir the pistachios, the cilantro, and remaining ¼ teaspoon black pepper into the cooked rice. Serve from the pot along with the chicken and its juices.

Healthy Kitchen Hack: Deanna likes experimenting with different spice, herb, and nut combos with this recipe depending on what she has on hand. Instead of cumin and pistachios, you can sub in equal amounts of ground cinnamon with almonds, dried rosemary with peanuts, dried thyme with walnuts, or create your own pairing!

PER SERVING: Calories: 421; Total Fat: 15g; Saturated Fat: 2g; Cholesterol: 83mg; Sodium: 218mg; Total Carbohydrates: 40g; Fiber: 4g; Protein: 33g

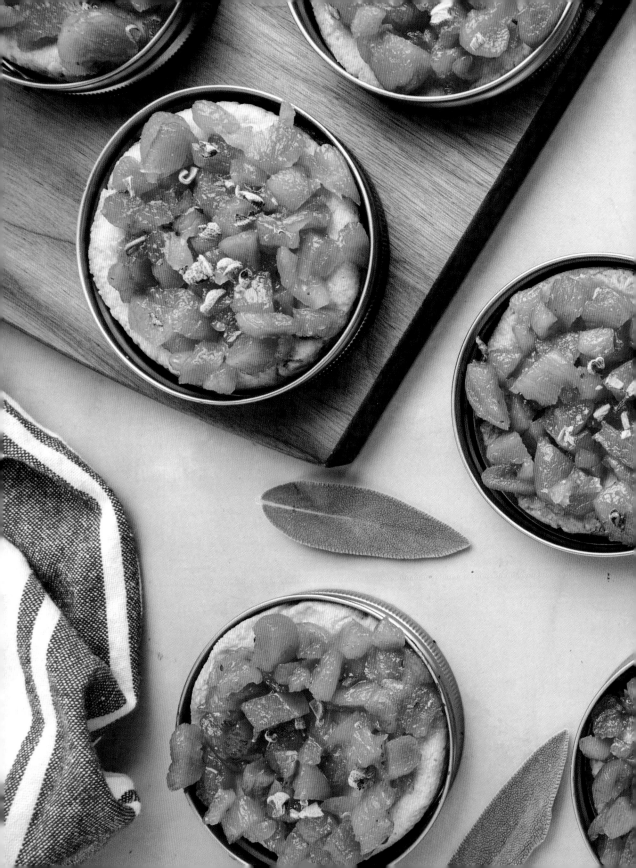

DESSERTS

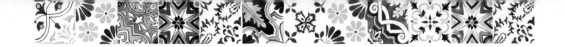

Coffee Yogurt
PANNA COTTA

SERVES 8   Prep time: 20 minutes, plus 2 hours chilling time

¼ cup very strong coffee or cold brew or 2 teaspoons instant coffee plus ¼ cup water

1 (7-gram) packet unflavored gelatin

2 cups plain whole-milk Greek yogurt or Homemade Yogurt (page 60)

1½ cups whole milk, divided

1 teaspoon vanilla extract

⅓ cup mild-flavored honey (see Tip)

¼ cup chopped roasted, salted pistachios or pumpkin seeds

Panna cotta is a dreamy Italian-style custard dessert that we enhanced with coffee for some brain benefits and flavor richness. Coffee has some of the highest concentration of antioxidants of any food or drink since it's sourced from coffee berries. Not only do these polyphenol antioxidants help stop brain damage from free radicals, but caffeine can also increase serotonin and stimulate the brain, perhaps improving memory. Serena likes to set the panna cotta in custard cups and then unmold onto dessert plates. You can also use pretty juice glasses to serve parfait-style.

Pour the cold or room-temperature coffee into a small bowl and sprinkle the gelatin over the top. Set aside to soften for 15 minutes.

Place 8 custard cups or small drinking glasses on a rimmed baking sheet or pan that will fit in the refrigerator.

In a large bowl, whisk together the yogurt, 1 cup milk, and the vanilla.

In a small saucepan, heat the remaining ½ cup milk and the honey over medium-low heat until it comes to a simmer, whisking just to combine. Remove from the heat and immediately whisk in the coffee-gelatin mixture. Pour over the yogurt mixture and whisk until completely combined.

Divide the mixture between the cups, then place the baking sheet in the refrigerator for at least 2 hours, or overnight to set.

continued on page 230

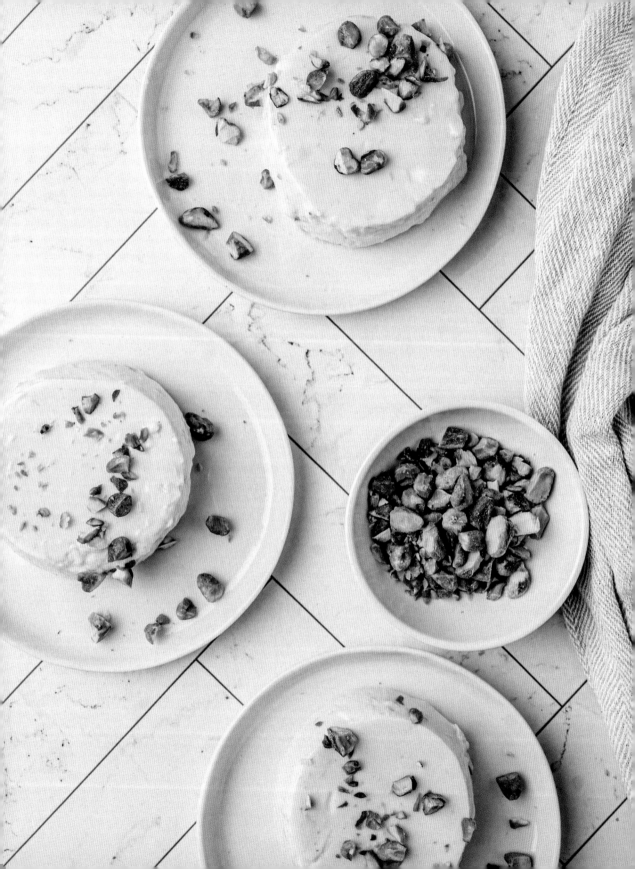

continued from page 228

To serve, sprinkle the tops of the cups with the pistachios. Or, to unmold, gently run a knife around each panna cotta to loosen from the cups, then turn upside-down onto a serving plate and sprinkle with pistachios.

Tip: Since this list of ingredients is short, you'll be able to taste each one. Use a mild, light-colored honey like wildflower or clover (the typical grocery store honey). If you use a darker honey (like raw-style or buckwheat), the flavor will be as strong as or even stronger than the coffee.

Healthy Kitchen Hack: We like to keep a jar of instant coffee in the cupboard to punch up the flavor (and brain benefits!) in recipes. Add a teaspoon to chocolate desserts to amp up the chocolate taste. Or add a teaspoon to your morning smoothie for a less expensive version of a bottled protein coffee drink—try it in our Chocolate-Tahini Power Shakes on page 34! In general, 1 teaspoon of most instant coffee granules averages about 60 mg of caffeine, bottle drinks range from 100 to 200 mg of caffeine, and an 8-ounce cup of coffee has 80 to 90 mg.

PER SERVING: Calories: 166; Total Fat: 7g; Saturated Fat: 3g; Cholesterol: 14mg; Sodium: 47mg; Total Carbohydrates: 18g; Fiber: 0g; Protein: 10g

Moroccan
SPICED HOT CHOCOLATE

SERVES 4 Prep time: 20 minutes ✳ Cook time: 10 minutes

Why not enjoy hot chocolate as a dessert? This luxurious-tasting drink is inspired by ras el hanout, the warming spice blend from Morocco, Tunisia, and Algeria, that is a mix of dozens of spices (see the Hack). Often used to flavor grains, vegetables, and meats (like our North African Spiced Yogurt Chicken on page 218), it also pairs perfectly with chocolate since sweet and spicy can complement each other while heightening the flavor and richness of the food. Enjoy this bevvy post meal or whenever you need a "brain break" to calm your mind and slow down a bit.

- 4 cups 2% milk
- 1 tablespoon sugar
- 1 small orange or mandarin orange
- 2 cinnamon sticks or ½ teaspoon ground cinnamon
- 3 cardamom pods, lightly crushed, or ¼ teaspoon ground cardamom
- ⅛ teaspoon cayenne pepper
- 3 ounces dark chocolate (70% or higher), broken up
- 1 teaspoon vanilla extract

In a medium saucepan, bring the milk to a simmer over medium heat. Remove the pan from the heat and whisk in the sugar. Using a vegetable peeler, peel off a 3-inch strip of orange rind and add it to the milk, along with the cinnamon, cardamom, and cayenne (save the remaining orange for another use). Let the spices steep for 15 minutes, then use a slotted spoon or mini wire mesh strainer to strain out the whole spices (if used) and orange peel.

Return the pan to medium-low heat and add the chocolate pieces. Heat until the chocolate melts, whisking occasionally, 3 to 5 minutes. Remove from the heat and stir in the vanilla. Serve immediately or chill and enjoy as an iced spiced chocolate milk.

Healthy Kitchen Hack: The spice mix of ras el hanout is often (but not limited to) a blend of paprika, cardamom, cumin, cloves, cinnamon, coriander, nutmeg, anise, ginger, peppercorns, and turmeric. Experiment and switch up the recipe above by swapping in or adding some of these spices for a unique cup of hot chocolate at every sitting.

PER SERVING: Calories: 263; Total Fat: 13g; Saturated Fat: 8g; Cholesterol: 21mg; Sodium: 118mg; Total Carbohydrates: 27g; Fiber: 2g; Protein: 10g

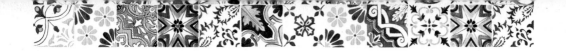

Dark Chocolate Chunk
SESAME SLAM COOKIES

MAKES ABOUT 18 COOKIES   Prep time: 15 minutes ✳ Cook time: 15 minutes

½ cup plus 1 tablespoon whole-wheat flour

½ cup all-purpose flour

½ teaspoon baking soda

½ teaspoon cornstarch

¼ teaspoon plus ⅛ teaspoon kosher or sea salt, divided

2 tablespoons sesame seeds, divided

¼ cup extra-virgin olive oil

2 tablespoons tahini

1 large egg

½ teaspoon vanilla extract

⅓ cup granulated sugar

⅓ cup packed brown sugar

2 ounces dark chocolate (70% or higher), chopped, or ¼ cup dark chocolate chips

❝

When I make cookies, I always want more! So I doubled this recipe and it worked great—and then I had more really, really good cookies.

JUDY FROM HAMEL, IL

A dessert a day can be a good thing for mental health, when you sit down and savor it fully. Just make sure to include some brain-boosting Mediterranean ingredients—and less sugar. One trick we use to make all our desserts taste sweet with less sugar is the balancing flavor of salt—here that salt on top hits your tongue first, so the following bite of sweet cookie tastes even sweeter! These cookies boast crispy outer edges and perfectly chewy insides. Then, there's the contrast of bittersweet smooth chocolate and toasty crunchy sesame seeds. Read on to discover how these "slam" cookies earned their name!

Arrange the oven racks in the upper-middle and lower-middle positions. Preheat the oven to 375°F. Line two large rimmed baking sheets with parchment paper.

In a medium bowl, whisk together the flours, baking soda, cornstarch, ¼ teaspoon salt, and 1 tablespoon sesame seeds. In a large bowl with an electric mixer or a stand mixer fitted with the whisk attachment, mix the oil, tahini, egg, and vanilla on medium speed until creamy, about 2 minutes. Add the sugars and mix to combine. Add the flour mixture and chocolate and mix until just combined, stopping once to scrape down the sides of the bowl.

Using a 1½-tablespoon scoop or measuring spoon, place dough portions on the prepared baking sheets about 3 inches apart. Using the bottom of a drinking glass or wet fingers, press down to flatten the cookies to about ¼ inch thickness and 2½ inches in diameter. Sprinkle the cookies with the remaining 1 tablespoon sesame seeds and remaining ⅛ teaspoon salt. Place a sheet on each oven rack and bake for 11 to 13 minutes, swapping and rotating the baking sheets halfway through, until the cookies no longer look moist.

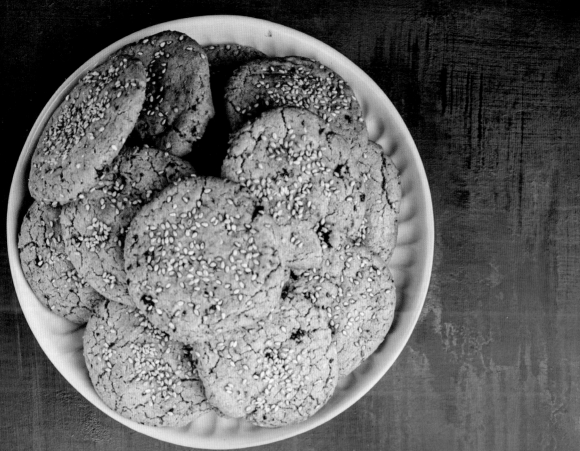

(Don't let them start to brown unless you want very crispy cookies.) Remove from the oven and immediately drop each baking sheet (from a height of about 8 inches) onto the counter 2 or 3 times—this "slamming" will help the cookies become chewier and more compact. Leave the cookies on the sheets for 5 minutes, then transfer to a wire rack to cool completely.

Healthy Kitchen Hack: If you prefer a chewy cookie to a puffy/cakey one in general, use the same ingredient swaps we used here to adapt any cookie recipe. Instead of shortening or solid butter, use an equal amount of olive oil. Use 2 to 3 tablespoons less flour. Use baking soda instead of baking powder, and add cornstarch. If your original recipe calls for chilling the dough, skip that step. Flatten cookie dough to ¼-inch thickness or less. Lastly, don't forget the "slam the pan" technique!

PER SERVING: (1 cookie):
Calories: 119; Total Fat: 6g;
Saturated Fat: 1g;
Cholesterol: 11mg;
Sodium: 61mg;
Total Carbohydrates: 15g;
Fiber: 1g; Protein: 2g

VANILLA YOGURT "SUNDAES"
with Honey-Fig Sauce

SERVES 4   Prep time: 25 minutes

¾ cup chopped dried figs (12 to 14)

2 teaspoons honey

2 teaspoons balsamic vinegar

¼ teaspoon dried thyme (optional)

2 cups 2% vanilla Greek yogurt

¼ cup chopped walnuts

4 teaspoons extra-virgin olive oil

¼ teaspoon kosher or sea salt

Warning: this honey fig sauce is so good, you may be tempted to eat it straight up with a spoon. Fortunately, the recipe makes extra. Figs are a classic staple in just about every Mediterranean country as the trees thrive in those climates. While fresh figs have a short early autumn season in America, dried figs are available year round and actually work best in this recipe. Plus they provide a healthy dose of fiber, and a growing body of research ties fiber consumption with a decreased risk of brain diseases. It may also help slow the aging of the brain.

In a large bowl, combine the chopped figs, honey, vinegar, and thyme, if using. Add ½ cup hot water, stir, and then let sit for 15 minutes.

Pour the softened fig mixture into a blender or food processor. Process until smooth.

To assemble the sundaes, spoon ½ cup yogurt into the bottoms of 4 tall glasses. Layer each sundae with 2 tablespoons fig sauce (you will need only half of the sauce for this recipe—store the remainder in an airtight container in the refrigerator for up to 1 week). Top each sundae with 1 tablespoon walnuts. Drizzle 1 teaspoon olive oil on top, add a pinch of salt, and serve.

Healthy Kitchen Hack: If you like a less sweet dessert or want to eat a sundae for breakfast, swap in plain Greek yogurt for the vanilla-flavored yogurt. Use your leftover fig sauce to make another round of sundaes or mix it into oatmeal, spread onto whole-grain toast, or spoon over grilled chicken.

PER SERVING: Calories: 263; Total Fat: 11g; Saturated Fat: 2g; Cholesterol: 6mg; Sodium: 202mg; Total Carbohydrates: 36g; Fiber: 3g; Protein: 8g

Slow Cooker
DARK CHOCOLATE FONDUE

SERVES 6   Prep time: 10 minutes   ✳   Cook time: 30 minutes

Sweet news! Researchers have found that a serving or two of dark chocolate may help with memory and reasoning. We enjoy its deep, rich flavor spiced with cinnamon, and also how well it pairs with so many Mediterranean fruits and nuts. When choosing dark chocolate, look for 70 percent cacao or higher to get the maximum antioxidant content and serve it with berries as one of your fruit choices whenever possible, as we do here, for even more brain-health benefits.

In a medium heat-safe glass bowl that will fit in a 6- or 7-quart slow cooker, whisk together the cocoa powder, honey, vanilla, cinnamon, and salt. Slowly whisk in the milk until well incorporated. Add the dark chocolate and place the bowl directly into the crock of the slow cooker. Cover and cook on high for 30 minutes. Whisk the fondue until the chocolate is smooth. If the chocolate is not fully melted, cook on low for about 15 minutes more. Reduce the setting to warm and serve directly from the slow cooker with the fruit; supply everyone with skewers for dipping.

Healthy Kitchen Hack: For an extra brain boost, a pop of color, and a yummy crunch, sprinkle pomegranate seeds (arils) and/or chopped nuts over your chocolate-dipped fruit. Pomegranates contain protective antioxidants, while nuts are packed with healthy monounsaturated fats, which may lower the risk of stroke. These "crunchies" also add fiber—in addition to the cocoa powder, which supplies 4 grams of gut-friendly fiber per serving!

½ cup unsweetened cocoa powder

¼ cup honey

2 teaspoons vanilla extract

¼ teaspoon ground cinnamon or smoked paprika

⅛ teaspoon kosher or sea salt

1 cup canned evaporated 2% milk

4 ounces dark chocolate (70% or higher), chopped

2 pints blackberries, raspberries, and/or strawberries (about 4 cups)

2 clementines, mandarins, or 1 orange, peeled and sectioned

12 fresh or dried figs

PER SERVING: (¼ cup fondue with fruit): Calories: 306; Total Fat: 11g; Saturated Fat: 5g; Cholesterol: 5mg; Sodium: 75mg; Total Carbohydrates: 51g; Fiber: 10g; Protein: 7g (Note: Nutritional values will vary depending on fruit used.)

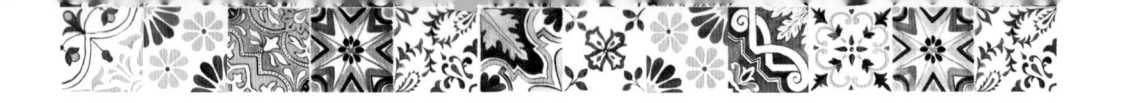

Mini APRICOT-SAGE TARTS

MAKES 8 MINI TARTS · Prep time: 15 minutes ❄ Cook time: 25 minutes

1¼ cups all-purpose flour

¼ cup sugar

1 large egg

½ teaspoon vanilla extract

10 fresh sage leaves, finely chopped, divided, plus more for garnish (optional)

5 tablespoons chilled unsalted butter, cut into small pieces

2 tablespoons apricot preserves

⅛ teaspoon kosher or sea salt

1 lemon

1½ cups finely chopped dried Mediterranean apricots (about 42 apricots)

Whipped cream or vanilla Greek yogurt, for serving (optional)

Using canning jar lids and rims as mini tart molds is one of Deanna's favorite baking hacks. Besides their bakery-quality appearance, these fruit and herb tarts also deliver big on nutrients thanks to the humble dried apricot, a quintessential Mediterranean fruit. Apricots contain magnesium, which can reduce headache occurrences, along with B vitamins that may help reduce the risk of depression.

Preheat the oven to 400°F. Cut parchment paper into circles to fit into eight 3½-inch metal canning jar lids with rims. Coat with cooking spray.

In a large bowl with an electric mixer or a stand mixer fitted with the paddle attachment, mix the flour, sugar, egg, vanilla, and half of the sage on low speed. Add the butter and mix until a sticky ball of dough forms.

Transfer the dough to a heavily floured surface and knead a few times. Divide the dough into 8 equal portions. Pat each portion with your hands or roll with a rolling pin into a 4-inch circle. Place each dough circle in a mason jar lid. Pat down and push the dough up the inside rim. Prick the bottom of each crust with a fork. Put the mason jar crusts on a large rimmed baking sheet and bake for about 20 minutes, until the crusts' edges start to turn golden brown. Set aside to cool slightly. (Keep the oven on.)

While the crusts bake, in a small pot, whisk together the apricot preserves, ½ cup water, and the salt. Using a Microplane or citrus zester, grate the zest from the lemon into the pot, then cut the lemon in half and squeeze in the juice; whisk together. Heat the mixture over medium heat until the preserves melt, about 1 minute. Mix in the dried apricots and cook until the apricots soften, 8 to 10 minutes. Remove from the heat and mix in the remaining sage.

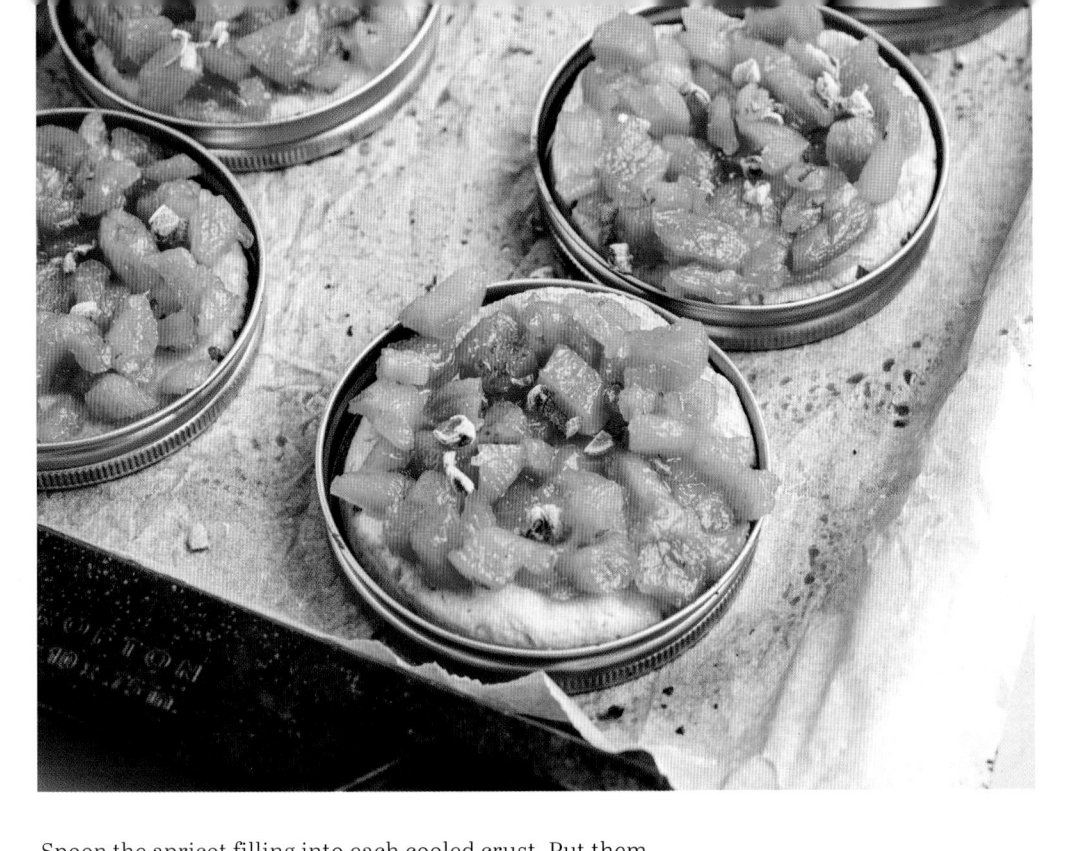

Spoon the apricot filling into each cooled crust. Put them back in the oven and bake for an additional 5 minutes, or until heated through. Remove the tarts from the oven and cool for 10 minutes. Before serving, remove the tarts from the lids and, if desired, serve each with a dollop of whipped cream or vanilla Greek yogurt and extra sage.

Healthy Kitchen Hack: While we adore this unique apricot-sage combo, depending on which fruit is in season, the frozen fruit you have on hand, or the dried fruit in your pantry, you can create endless fruit + herb fillings for these mini tarts. Try:

> Fresh, frozen, or dried cherries + fresh basil

> Fresh or frozen berries + fresh mint

> Fresh or frozen peaches + fresh thyme

> Fresh or canned pears + fresh rosemary

> *My husband loved these, and I added a sliver of sage to the top of each tart for presentation.*
>
> TONI FROM
> INDIO, CA

PER SERVING: (1 tart without topping): Calories: 245; Total Fat: 8g; Saturated Fat: 5g; Cholesterol: 42mg; Sodium: 45mg; Total Carbohydrates: 41g; Fiber: 3g; Protein: 4g

Cherry-Pomegranate
RISOTTO PUDDING

SERVES 6   Prep time: 10 minutes   ✳ Cook time: 2½ hours

3 cups 2% milk

⅔ cup uncooked Arborio (risotto) rice or other short-grain rice

3 tablespoons sugar

¼ teaspoon kosher or sea salt

1 cup frozen cherries, thawed and chopped, or ⅓ cup chopped dried cherries

1 teaspoon vanilla extract

2 tablespoons pomegranate molasses (see Hack on page 177) or honey

¼ cup chopped pistachios

Serena found making rice pudding in the slow cooker to be a revelation as there's no standing over the stove constantly stirring a pot. This stunningly easy-to-make, comforting rice pudding can be served as dessert or a hearty snack—or even for breakfast. The combo of cherry, pomegranate, and pistachio is decidedly Mediterranean and decidedly good for lifting your mood!

Spray the slow cooker insert with cooking spray. Add the milk, ½ cup water, rice, sugar, and salt and whisk well to combine. Cover and cook on low for 2½ hours, or until the rice is soft and the liquid has thickened, stirring each hour during cooking. Turn off the heat and mix in the cherries and vanilla. Let sit uncovered for 10 minutes (or let cool completely and chill before serving). Spoon into serving cups, drizzle with the pomegranate molasses, top with the pistachios, and serve.

Healthy Kitchen Hack: Mix up your Mediterranean pudding recipe with these fruit-nut-spice-herb combos:

> Prunes + walnuts + fresh thyme

> Dried apricots + sesame seeds + ground ginger

> Fresh or frozen peaches/nectarines + almonds + ground nutmeg

> Oranges + pecans + ground cinnamon

PER SERVING: Calories: 237, Total Fat: 5g; Saturated Fat: 2g; Cholesterol: 10mg; Sodium: 139mg; Total Carbohydrates: 43g; Fiber: 1g; Protein: 7g

SEMOLINA CAKE
with Candied Lemon Slices

SERVES 16 Prep time: 45 minutes, plus 2 hours resting ❋ Cook time: 30 minutes

Surprisingly light in texture for an olive oil cake, this one is soaked in a bright lemon syrup and is inspired by similar desserts from many countries touched by the Mediterranean sun: Libyan basbousa, Lebanese sfouf, Italian torta di semolino, Greek revani, and Turkish tishpishti, which also has roots in Spain and Syria. Common among all these cakes are the ingredients semolina, lemon, almonds, sugar, milk, and lots of oil or butter, with variations also including rose water, sesame seeds, other nuts, cinnamon, raisins, ricotta cheese, honey, dried fruits, and even rum. Feel free to embellish this sweet treat in any way you and your brain would love!

1 cup semolina flour or farina (see Hack)

1 cup plain whole-milk Greek yogurt or Homemade Yogurt (page 60)

½ cup extra-virgin olive oil

½ cup whole-wheat flour

2 teaspoons baking powder

½ teaspoon baking soda

½ teaspoon kosher or sea salt

2 lemons

1¼ cups sugar, divided

2 large eggs

Preheat the oven to 350°F. Heavily coat a 9-inch square baking pan with cooking spray.

In a medium bowl, mix together the semolina, yogurt, and oil and set aside to hydrate for 30 minutes (this will help achieve a moist and uniform texture in the cake).

In another medium bowl, whisk together the flour, baking powder, baking soda, and salt.

Using a Microplane or citrus zester, grate the zest from one lemon into the bowl of a stand mixer. Cut the lemon in half and squeeze 2 tablespoons juice into a small bowl and set aside; reserve the remaining lemon half.

Add ½ cup sugar and the eggs to the bowl with the lemon zest. Using the whisk attachment, beat until the mixture has lightened in color, about 2 minutes. Add the yogurt mixture and whisk well. Add the flour mixture and whisk just to combine. Pour into the prepared pan and, using a silicone spatula, smooth it out evenly.

continued on page 240

continued from page 239

Bake for 25 to 30 minutes, until a toothpick inserted in the center comes out with just a few crumbs. Let cool for only 10 minutes in the pan on a wire rack.

While the cake bakes (or the day before), slice the remaining lemon half and the other whole lemon into very thin slices (⅛ to ¼ inch thick). In a large skillet, combine ¾ cup water and the remaining ¾ cup sugar and heat over medium-low heat, stirring until the sugar dissolves. Add the lemon slices in a single layer and bring just to a simmer (when a few bubbles pop occasionally). Cook for 30 minutes, or until lemon skin is slightly translucent, flipping the lemon slices every 8 to 10 minutes. Turn off the heat. Transfer the slices to a sheet of parchment paper, letting excess syrup drip off and using a butter knife to gently scrape off any remaining. Let the slices dry for as long as possible before topping the cake, at least 2 hours. Reserve the syrup in the skillet.

After the cake cools for 10 minutes, poke holes in the cake at 1-inch intervals with a toothpick. Whisk the reserved lemon juice into the lemon syrup in the skillet and immediately pour over the cake. Let the cake sit for at least 2 hours before cutting.

Before serving, top the cake with the candied lemon slices. (You may have extra lemon slices to enjoy as candy!)

Tip: Some of the steps in this cake may seem a little fussy, but they are worth it to achieve the very best cake texture and taste! The candied lemon slices can be made the day before; let them dry for up to 24 hours on the counter before transferring (on the parchment paper) to an airtight container.

66

I made this cake with semolina and then made it with Cream of Wheat. I liked the texture of the Cream of Wheat version better, but both would be a special treat in a lunch box or on a picnic. The taste is reminiscent of traditional Italian Easter grain pie.

MARIA FROM
WESTLAKE VILLAGE, CA

PER SERVING: Calories: 199; Total Fat: 9g; Saturated Fat: 2g; Cholesterol: 26mg; Sodium: 95mg; Total Carbohydrates: 28g; Fiber: 1g; Protein: 4g

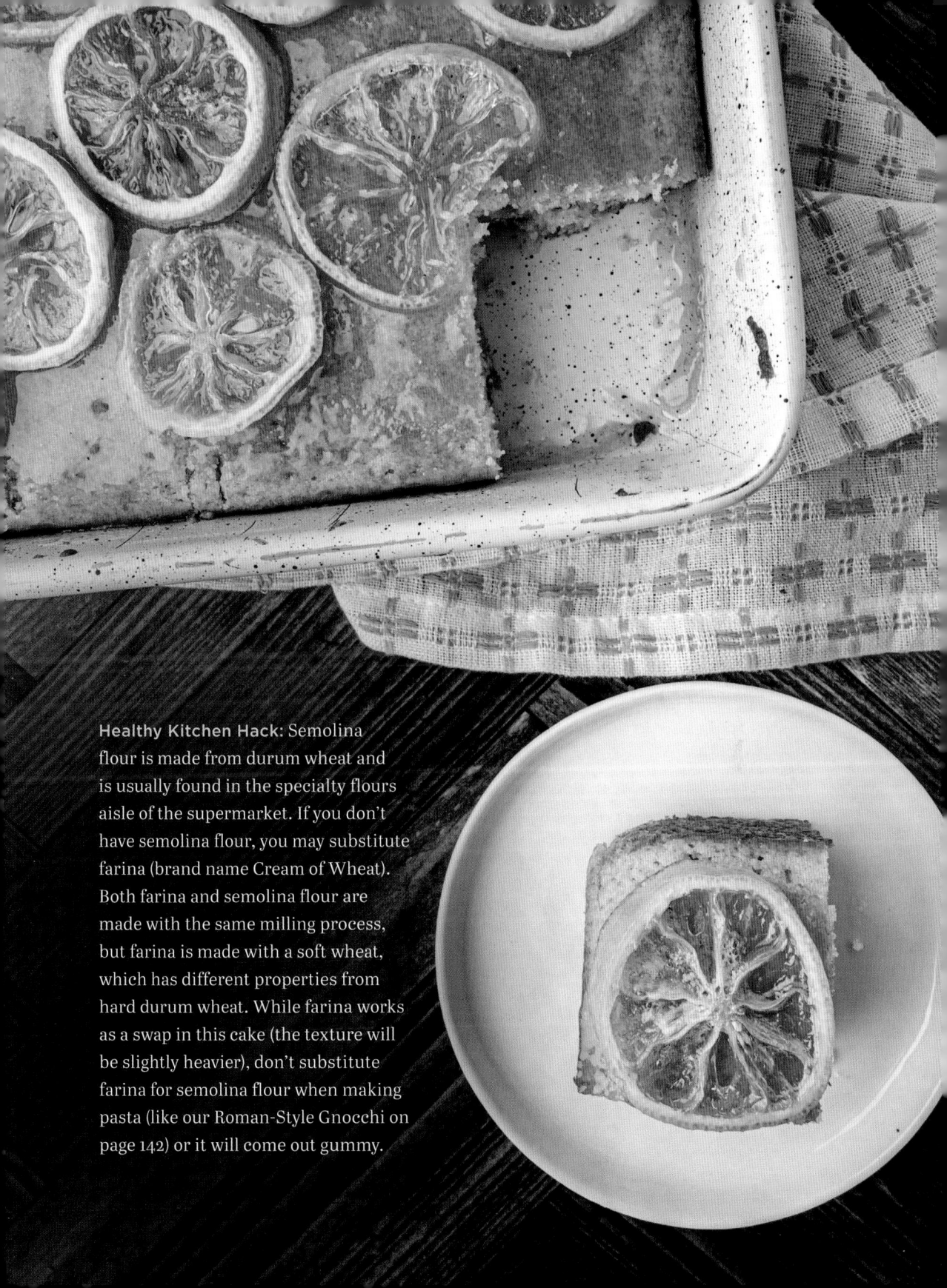

Healthy Kitchen Hack: Semolina flour is made from durum wheat and is usually found in the specialty flours aisle of the supermarket. If you don't have semolina flour, you may substitute farina (brand name Cream of Wheat). Both farina and semolina flour are made with the same milling process, but farina is made with a soft wheat, which has different properties from hard durum wheat. While farina works as a swap in this cake (the texture will be slightly heavier), don't substitute farina for semolina flour when making pasta (like our Roman-Style Gnocchi on page 142) or it will come out gummy.

RECILE GUIDE *for* SPECIAL DIETS

RECIPE GUIDE *for* SPECIAL DIETS

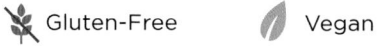

- 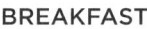 Dairy-Free
- Egg-Free
- Gluten-Free
- Nut-Free
- Vegetarian
- Vegan

	Dairy-Free	Egg-Free	Gluten-Free	Nut-Free	Vegetarian	Vegan
BREAKFAST						
Good Mood Mango-Cilantro Smoothies		●	●	●	●	
Smashed Cannellini and Avocado Toast with Za'atar	●	●		●	●	●
Shakshuka Scrambled Eggs with Chiles				●	●	
Chocolate-Tahini Power Shakes		●	●	●	●	
Cheesy Spinach and Egg Mug Scrambles with a Kick			●	●	●	
Mediterranean Sun Gold Granola	●	●	●	●	●	
On-the-Go Breakfast Flatbread Wraps		●		●	●	
Olive Oil Berry Breakfast Cake			●	●	●	
Nutmeg Oatmeal Custard			●	●	●	
SMALL PLATES & SNACKS						
Honey-Turmeric Salted Peanuts	●	●	●		●	
Marvelous Mediterranean Olives	●	●	●	●	●	●
Sweet and Smoky Chickpea Crunchies	●	●	●	●	●	●
North African Sweet Hot Pepper Pickles	●	●	●	●	●	●
Walnut and Herb-Crusted Baked Goat Cheese		●			●	
Baby Lima Bean Dip with Parsley and Pomegranate	●	●	●	●	●	●
Cumin-Sesame Chickpea Crackers	●	●	●	●	●	●
Homemade Yogurt		●	●	●	●	

SALADS

	Dairy-Free	Egg-Free	Gluten-Free	Nut-Free	Vegetarian	Vegan
Berry Smart Seeded Dressing over Greens		●	●		●	
Creamy Cucumber Salad with Sesame Dressing		●	●	●	●	
September Apple-Celery Salad		●	●		●	
Roasted Orange, Asparagus, and Parmesan Salad		●	●	●	●	
Melon and Prosciutto Panzanella	●	●		●		
Green Couscous Lettuce Scoops		●			●	
Black Lentil Salad with Toasted Cumin	●		●	●	●	
Spicy Green Bean and Potato Salad	●	●	●		●	●

SIDES

	Dairy-Free	Egg-Free	Gluten-Free	Nut-Free	Vegetarian	Vegan
Black Pepper and Coffee Roasted Carrots	●	●	●	●	●	
Magical Olive Oil Potato Hash	●	●	●	●	●	●
Brussels Sprout Sauté with Hazelnuts		●	●		●	
Pan-Roasted Mushrooms in Wine and Thyme	●	●	●	●	●	●
Corn, Cilantro, and Pomegranate Medley	●	●	●			
Roasted Radishes with Green Olive Salsa Verde	●	●	●	●	●	●
Sautéed Greens with Honey-Tahini Sauce	●	●	●	●		
Roasted Potatoes and Beets with Herbed Ricotta		●	●	●	●	

SOUPS

	Dairy-Free	Egg-Free	Gluten-Free	Nut-Free	Vegetarian	Vegan
Spiced Tomato Soup with Fried Halloumi		●	●	●	●	
Cozy "Cream" of Mushroom Soup		●				
Spicy Turmeric Chicken Minestrone Soup		●		●		
Tunisian Peanut-Lentil Soup	●	●	●			●
Ginger Butternut Squash Soup with Tahini and Toasted Seeds		●	●	●	●	
Stracciatella Soup with Chicken and Spinach			●	●		
Turkish White Bean Soup with Aleppo Pepper	●	●	●	●	●	●
Cream of Artichoke Soup with Goat Cheese Pita Toasts		●	●	●	●	

SANDWICHES & PIZZA

Dish	🥛	🚫🥛	🌾	🥜	🥕	🌿
Roasted Veggie and Beet Hummus Sandwiches	●	●		●	●	●
Crispy Eggplant Pitas with Mediterranean Mayo				●	●	
Chef Lorenzo's Snack Sandwiches	●	●				
Provençal Grilled Cheese with Walnut Mustard Spread		●			●	
Smarter Pizza Dough		●			●	
Caprese Salad Pizza		●		●	●	
Three-Cheese Pizza with Sweet Potato		●		●	●	
Scallion Flatbread with Mozzarella and Olives				●	●	

PASTA

Dish	🥛	🚫🥛	🌾	🥜	🥕	🌿
Speedy Pesto Sauce		●	●		●	
Pasta Ceci e Broccolini	●	●		●		●
Smart and Spicy Summer Spaghetti		●		●	●	
Fettuccine with Prosciutto, Prunes, and Black Pepper		●		●		
Save-the-Day Slow Cooker Lasagna		●		●		
Marinated Eggplant Fusilli with Feta and Mint		●		●	●	
Oven-Baked Gnocchi with Lemon–Black Pepper Sauce		●		●		
Roman-Style Gnocchi with Olives and Thyme				●	●	
Shortcut Homemade Ravioli					●	
Mushroom Pastitsio "Baked" Pasta				●	●	

VEG MAIN DISHES

Dish	🥛	🚫🥛	🌾	🥜	🥕	🌿
Speedy Paella with Cauliflower Rice	●	●	●	●	●	●
Artichoke Rainbow Veggie Bake				●	●	
Green Falafel Fritters with Red Pepper Sauce		●			●	
One-Pot Spanish Beans and Barley	●	●			●	●
Ratatouille with Socca	●	●	●	●	●	●
7-Spice Mushroom Bulgur Stuffed Zucchini		●				
Mushroom Daube	●	●		●	●	●
Crisp Corn Cakes with Goat Cheese and Tomatoes				●	●	
Egyptian Koshari with Sautéed Onions	●	●		●	●	●
Potato and Cheese Bourekas				●	●	
Slow Cooker Baked Potatoes with Mediterranean Toppers		●	●	●	●	
Sweet Potato Farro Bowls with Pomegranate Molasses	●	●			●	

SEAFOOD	🥛	🥚	🌾	🥜	🥕	🌿
Quick Fish with Walnut-Arugula Pesto		●	●			
Easiest Broiled Shrimp	●	●	●	●		
Roasted Salmon and Avocado Fattoush	●	●				
Grilled Fish with Almond Honey Mustard Sauce	●	●	●			
Sizzling Shrimp and Peppers with Cilantro	●	●	●			
Chermoula Tuna Burgers				●		
Crispy Za'atar Tilapia with Orange Slices	●	●	●			
Broiled Trout with Coriander and Cilantro		●	●	●		
Scallops Fra Diavolo	●	●	●			
Clam and Leek Mini Pot Pies				●		
Potato Tortilla with Mackerel and Peppers	●		●	●		
Puttanesca Fish Stew	●	●	●	●		

MEAT & CHICKEN	🥛	🥚	🌾	🥜	🥕	🌿
Steak au Poivre with Herbes de Provence Potato Wedges	●	●	●	●		
Lebanese Spiced Cabbage Rolls with Rice	●	●	●	●		
Honey-Tahini Pork Tenderloin	●	●	●	●		
Palestinian Kafta with Lots of Parsley	●			●		
Chicken Kebabs with Grapes and Olives	●	●	●	●		
Pan-Fried Parmesan-Pecan Chicken		●	●			
North African Spiced Yogurt Chicken		●	●	●		
Braised Chicken Kapama over Orzo		●		●		
Blueberry Turkey Panzanella		●				
Pomegranate Chicken with Turmeric Pistachio Rice	●	●	●			

DESSERTS	🥛	🥚	🌾	🥜	🥕	🌿
Coffee Yogurt Panna Cotta		●	●			
Moroccan Spiced Hot Chocolate		●		●	●	
Dark Chocolate Chunk Sesame Slam Cookies	●			●	●	
Vanilla Yogurt "Sundaes" with Honey-Fig Sauce		●				
Slow Cooker Dark Chocolate Fondue		●	●	●	●	
Mini Apricot-Sage Tarts				●	●	
Cherry-Pomegranate Risotto Pudding		●	●		●	
Semolina Cake with Candied Lemon Slices				●	●	

FIVE-DAY MEAL PLANS

MONDAY	Gluten-Free	Vegetarian	Seafood 4x week	Meatless Monday
Breakfast	Olive Oil Berry Breakfast Cake 43 (made on the weekend), berries, coffee	Olive Oil Berry Breakfast Cake 43 (made on the weekend), berries, coffee	Olive Oil Berry Breakfast Cake 43 (made on the weekend), berries, coffee	Olive Oil Berry Breakfast Cake 43 (made on the weekend), berries, coffee
Lunch	Stracciatella Soup with Chicken and Spinach 106, seeded gluten-free bread slices	Turkish White Bean Soup with Aleppo Pepper 107, seeded bread slices	Stracciatella Soup with Chicken and Spinach 106, seeded bread slices	Turkish White Bean Soup with Aleppo Pepper 107, seeded bread slices
Snack	Homemade Yogurt 60 (made on the weekend to use all week) with veggies, gluten-free crackers	Homemade Yogurt 60 (made on the weekend to use all week) with veggies, crackers	Homemade Yogurt 60 (made on the weekend to use all week) with veggies, crackers	Homemade Yogurt 60 (made on the weekend to use all week) with veggies, crackers
Dinner	Mushroom Pastitsio "Baked" Pasta 148 (made with gluten-free pasta and flour), raw vegetables with Mediterranean Mayo 114	Mushroom Pastitsio "Baked" Pasta 148, raw vegetables with Mediterranean Mayo 114	Sizzling Shrimp and Peppers with Cilantro 186, raw vegetables with Mediterranean Mayo 114	Mushroom Pastitsio "Baked" Pasta 148, raw vegetables with Mediterranean Mayo 114
Dessert	Moroccan Spiced Hot Chocolate 231	Moroccan Spiced Hot Chocolate 231	Moroccan Spiced Hot Chocolate 231	Moroccan Spiced Hot Chocolate 231

TUESDAY	Gluten-Free	Vegetarian	Seafood 4x week	Meatless Monday
Breakfast	Leftover Olive Oil Berry Breakfast Cake, fruit, cafe latte	Leftover Olive Oil Berry Breakfast Cake, fruit, cafe latte	Leftover Olive Oil Berry Breakfast Cake, fruit, cafe latte	Leftover Olive Oil Berry Breakfast Cake, fruit, cafe latte
Lunch	Sweet Potato Farro Bowls with Pomegranate Molasses 176 (made with quinoa)	Sweet Potato Farro Bowls with Pomegranate Molasses 176	Sweet Potato Farro Bowls with Pomegranate Molasses 176	Sweet Potato Farro Bowls with Pomegranate Molasses 176
Snack	Cumin-Sesame Chickpea Crackers 58, cheese, raw veggies	Cumin-Sesame Chickpea Crackers 58, cheese, raw veggies	Cumin-Sesame Chickpea Crackers 58, cheese, raw veggies	Cumin-Sesame Chickpea Crackers 58, cheese, raw veggies
Dinner	Quick Fish with Walnut-Arugula Pesto 180 on instant brown rice, broccoli	Slow Cooker Baked Potatoes with Mediterranean Toppers 174	Quick Fish with Walnut-Arugula Pesto 180 on couscous, broccoli	Quick Fish with Walnut-Arugula Pesto 180 on couscous, broccoli
Dessert	A few pieces of dark chocolate	A few pieces of dark chocolate	A few pieces of dark chocolate	A few pieces of dark chocolate

WEDNESDAY	Gluten-Free	Vegetarian	Seafood 4x week	Meatless Monday
Breakfast	On-the-Go Breakfast Flatbread Wraps 40 (made with gluten-free flatbread)	On-the-Go Breakfast Flatbread Wraps 40	On-the-Go Breakfast Flatbread Wraps 40	On-the-Go Breakfast Flatbread Wraps 40
Lunch	Low-sodium canned tomato soup with leftover filling from Breakfast Flatbread stirred in, canned tuna on gluten-free crackers	Low-sodium canned tomato soup with leftover filling from Breakfast Flatbread stirred in, cheese on whole-grain crackers	Low-sodium canned tomato soup with leftover filling from Breakfast Flatbread stirred in, canned tuna on whole-grain crackers	Low-sodium canned tomato soup with leftover filling from Breakfast Flatbread stirred in, canned tuna on whole-grain crackers

FRIDAY	Gluten-Free	Vegetarian	Seafood 4x week	Meatless Monday
Breakfast	Good Mood Mango-Cilantro Smoothies 28, gluten-free toast	Good Mood Mango-Cilantro Smoothies 28, whole-grain toast	Good Mood Mango-Cilantro Smoothies 28, whole-grain toast	Good Mood Mango-Cilantro Smoothies 28, whole-grain toast
Lunch	Black Lentil Salad with Toasted Cumin 75 with 2 extra hard-boiled eggs	Black Lentil Salad with Toasted Cumin 75 with 2 extra hard-boiled eggs	Black Lentil Salad with Toasted Cumin 75 with 2 extra hard-boiled eggs	Black Lentil Salad with Toasted Cumin 75 with 2 extra hard-boiled eggs
Snack	Walnut and Herb-Crusted Baked Goat Cheese 54 with gluten-free crackers, wine or sparkling grape juice	Walnut and Herb-Crusted Baked Goat Cheese 54, wine or sparkling grape juice	Walnut and Herb-Crusted Baked Goat Cheese 54, wine or sparkling grape juice	Walnut and Herb-Crusted Baked Goat Cheese 54, wine or sparkling grape juice
Dinner	Puttanesca Fish Stew 201, gluten-free bread, green salad with leftover fennel and capers from stew	Roman-Style Gnocchi with Olives and Thyme 144, whole-grain bread, green salad with leftover olives from gnocchi	Puttanesca Fish Stew 201, whole-grain bread, green salad with leftover fennel and capers from stew	Puttanesca Fish Stew 201, whole-grain bread, green salad with leftover fennel and capers from stew
Dessert	Slow Cooker Dark Chocolate Fondue 235	Slow Cooker Dark Chocolate Fondue 235	Slow Cooker Dark Chocolate Fondue 235	Slow Cooker Dark Chocolate Fondue 235

THURSDAY	Gluten-Free	Vegetarian	Seafood 4x week	Meatless Monday
Breakfast	Cheesy Spinach and Egg Mug Scrambles with a Berry Kick 37, berries	Cheesy Spinach and Egg Mug Scrambles with a Berry Kick 37, berries	Cheesy Spinach and Egg Mug Scrambles with a Berry Kick 37, berries	Cheesy Spinach and Egg Mug Scrambles with a Berry Kick 37, berries
Lunch	Leftover Honey-Tahini Pork Tenderloin, gluten-free pita bread, fruit	Leftover Artichoke Rainbow Veggie Bake, pita bread, fruit	Leftover Palestinian Kafta with Lots of Parsley, pita bread, fruit	Leftover Palestinian Kafta with Lots of Parsley, pita bread, fruit
Snack	North African Sweet Hot Pepper Pickles 53 (made day before) with cheese	North African Sweet Hot Pepper Pickles 53 (made day before) with cheese	North African Sweet Hot Pepper Pickles 53 (made day before) with cheese	North African Sweet Hot Pepper Pickles 53 (made day before) with cheese
Dinner	Braised Chicken Kapama over Orzo 220 (use gluten-free orzo or other gluten-free small pasta shape), cabbage slaw with leftover Berry Smart Seeded Dressing	Pasta Ceci e Broccolini 131, cabbage slaw with leftover Berry Smart Seeded Dressing	Braised Chicken Kapama over Orzo 220, cabbage slaw with leftover Berry Smart Seeded Dressing	Braised Chicken Kapama over Orzo 220, cabbage slaw with leftover Berry Smart Seeded Dressing
Dessert	Vanilla Yogurt "Sundaes" with Honey-Fig Sauce 234	Vanilla Yogurt "Sundaes" with Honey-Fig Sauce 234	Vanilla Yogurt "Sundaes" with Honey-Fig Sauce 234	Vanilla Yogurt "Sundaes" with Honey-Fig Sauce 234

	Gluten-Free	Vegetarian	Seafood 4x week	Meatless Monday
Snack	Honey-Turmeric Salted Peanuts 48	Honey-Turmeric Salted Peanuts 48	Honey-Turmeric Salted Peanuts 48	Honey-Turmeric Salted Peanuts 48
Dinner	Honey-Tahini Pork Tenderloin 209, gluten-free pita bread, Berry Smart Seeded Dressing over Greens 64 (save half the dressing)	Artichoke Rainbow Veggie Bake 154, Berry Smart Seeded Dressing over Greens 64 (save half the dressing)	Palestinian Kafta with Lots of Parsley 212, pita bread, Berry Smart Seeded Dressing over Greens 64 (save half the dressing)	Palestinian Kafta with Lots of Parsley 212, pita bread, Berry Smart Seeded Dressing over Greens 64 (save half the dressing)
Dessert	Cherry-Pomegranate Risotto Pudding 238	Cherry-Pomegranate Risotto Pudding 238	Cherry-Pomegranate Risotto Pudding 238	Cherry-Pomegranate Risotto Pudding 238

SELECTED BIBLIOGRAPHY

Chauhan, Abha, and Ved Chauhan. "Beneficial Effects of Walnuts on Cognition and Brain Health." *Nutrients* 12, no. 2 (2020): 550. https://doi.org/10.3390/nu12020550.

Daly, Trevor, Marvin A. Jiwan, Nora M. O'Brien, and S. Aisling Aherne. "Carotenoid Content of Commonly Consumed Herbs and Assessment of Their Bioaccessibility Using an *In Vitro* Digestion Model." *Plant Foods for Human Nutrition* 65 (2010): 164–169. https://doi.org/10.1007/s11130-010-0167-3.

Esnafoğlu, Erman, and Elif Yaman. "Vitamin B12, Folic Acid, Homocysteine and Vitamin D Levels in Children and Adolescents with Obsessive Compulsive Disorder." *Psychiatry Research* 254 (2017): 232–237. https://doi.org/10.1016/j.psychres.2017.04.032.

Foshati, Sahar, Ahmad Ghanizadeh, and Masoumeh Akhlaghi. "Extra-Virgin Olive Oil Improves Depression Symptoms without Affecting Salivary Cortisol and Brain-Derived Neurotrophic Factor in Patients with Major Depression: A Double-Blind Randomized Controlled Trial." *Journal of the Academy of Nutrition and Dietetics* 122, no. 2 (2022): 284–297.e1. https://doi.org/10.1016/j.jand.2021.07.016.

Frances, Heather M., Richard J. Stevenson, Jaime R. Chambers, Dolly Gupta, Brooklyn Newey, and Chai K. Lim. "A Brief Diet Intervention Can Reduce Symptoms of Depression in Young Adults —A Randomised Controlled Trial." *PLOS One* (2019). https://doi.org/10.1371/journal.pone.0222768.

Juton, Charlotte, Paula Berruezo, Luis Rajmil, Carles Lerin, Montserrat Fíto, Clara Homs, Genís Según, Santiago F. Gómez, and Helmut Schröder. "Prospective Association between Adherence to the Mediterranean Diet Related Quality of Life in Spanish Children." *Nutrients* 14 (2022): 5304. https://doi.org/10.3390/nu14245304.

Kantak, Pranish A., Dylan N. Bobrow, and John G. Nyby. "Obsessive-Compulsive-Like Behaviors in House Mice Are Attenuated by a Probiotic (*Lactobacillus rhamnosus GG*)." *Behavioral Pharmacology* 25, no. 1 (2014): 71–79. https://doi.org/10.1097/fbp.0000000000000013.

Keenan, Tiarnán D., Elvira Agrón, Julie A. Mares, Traci E. Clemons, Freekje van Asten, Anand Swaroop, Emily Y. Chew, and AREDS and AREDS2 Research Groups. "Adherence to a Mediterranean Diet and Cognitive Function in the Age-Related Eye Disease Studies 1 & 2." *Alzheimer's & Dementia* 16, no. 6 (2020): 831–842. https://doi.org/10.1002/alz.12077.

Khasnavis, Saurabh, and Kalipada Pahan. "Cinnamon Treatment Upregulates Neuroprotective Proteins Parkin and DJ-1 and Protects Dopaminergic Neurons in a Mouse Model of Parkinson's Disease." *Journal of Neuroimmune Pharmacology* 9 (2014): 569–581. https://doi.org/10.1007/s11481-014-9552-2.

Kim, Chong-Su, and Dong-Mi Shin. "Probiotic Food Consumption Is Associated with Lower Severity and Prevalence of Depression: A Nationwide Cross-Sectional Study." *Nutrition* 63–64 (2019): 169–174. https://doi.org/10.1016/j.nut.2019.02.007.

Liu, Cheng-Hui, Xian-Le Bu, Jun Wang, Tao Zhang, Yang Xiang, Lin-Lin Shen, Qing-Hua Wang, Bo Deng, Xin Wang, Chi Zhu, Xiu-Qing Yao, et al. "The Associations between a Capsaicin-Rich Diet and Blood Amyloid-Levels and Cognitive Function." *Journal of Alzheimer's Disease* 52, no. 3 (2016): 1081–1088. https://doi.org/10.3233/jad-151079.

Lu, Ping, Cheng-Hai Zhang, Lawrence M. Lifshitz, and Ronghua ZhuGe. "Extraoral Bitter Taste Receptors in Health and Disease." *Journal of General Physiology* 149, no. 2 (2017): 181–197. https://doi.org/10.1085/jgp.201611637.

Martínez-Lapiscina, Elena H., P. Clavero, E. Toledo, B. San Julian, A. Sanchez-Tainta, D. Corella, R. M. Lamuela-Raventos, J. A. Martinez, and M. Á. Martinez-Gonzalez. "Virgin Olive Oil Supplementation and Long-Term Cognition: The PREDIMED-NAVARRA Randomized Trial." *Journal of Nutrition, Health and Aging* 17, no. 6 (2013): 544–552. https://doi.org/10.1007/s12603-013-0027-6.

McEvoy, Claire T., Heidi Guyer, Kenneth M. Langa, and Kristine Yaffe. "Neuroprotective Diets Are Associated with Better Cognitive Function: The Health and Retirement Study." *Journal of the American Geriatric Society* 65, no. 8 (2017): 1857–1862. https://doi.org/10.1111/jgs.14922.

Morris, Martha Clare, Christy C. Tangney, Yamin Wang, Frank M. Sacks, Lisa L. Barnes, David A. Bennett, and Neelum T. Aggarwal. "MIND Diet Slows Cognitive Decline with Aging." *Alzheimer's and Dementia* 11, no. 9 (2015): 1015–1022. https://doi.org/10.1016/j.jalz.2015.04.011.

Pan, Enhui, Xiao-an Zhang, Zhen Huang, Christine E. Tinberg, Stephen J. Lippard, and James O. McNamara. "Vesicular Zinc Promotes Presynaptic and Inhibits Postsynaptic Long-Term Potentiation of Mossy Fiber-CA3 Synapse." *Neuron* 71, no. 6 (2011): 1116–1126. https://doi.org/10.1016/j.neuron.2011.07.019.

Ren, Bo, Tian Yuan, Zhijun Diao, Chenxi Zhang, Zhigang Liua, and Xuebo Liu. "Protective Effects of Sesamol on Systemic Oxidative Stress-Induced Cognitive Impairments via Regulation of Nrf2/Keap1 Pathway." *Food & Function* 9 (2018): 5912–5924. https://doi.org/10.1039/C8FO01436A.

Renzi-Hammond, Lisa M., Emily R. Bovier, Laura M. Fletcher, L. Stephen Miller, Catherine M. Mewborn, Cutter A. Lindbergh, Jeffrey H. Baxter, and Billy R. Hammond. "Effects of a Lutein and Zeaxanthin Intervention on Cognitive Function: A Randomized, Double-Masked, Placebo-Controlled Trial of Younger Healthy Adults." *Nutrients* 9, no. 11 (2017): 1246. https://doi.org/10.3390/nu9111246.

Romero Cabrera, Angel Julio. "Zinc, Aging, and Immunosenescence: An Overview." *Pathobiology of Aging and Age-related Diseases* 5, no. 1 (2015). https://doi.org/10.3402/pba.v5.25592.

Saenghong, Naritsara, Jintanaporn Wattanathorn, Supaporn Muchimapura, Terdthai Tongun, Nawanant Piyavhatkul, Chuleratana Banchonglikitkul, and Tanwarat Kajsongkram. "*Zingiber officinale* Improves Cognitive Function of the Middle-Aged Healthy Women." *Evidence-Based Complementary Alternative Medicine* 2012 (2012): 383062. https://doi.org/10.1155/2012/383062.

Saunders, Erika F.H., Dahlia Mukherjee, Tiffany Myers, Emily Wasserman, Ahmad Hameed, Venkatesh Bassappa Krishnamurthy, Beth MacIntosh, Anthony Domenichiello, Christopher E. Ramsden, and Ming Wang. "Adjunctive Dietary Intervention for Bipolar Disorder: A Randomized, Controlled, Parallel-Group, Modified Double-Blinded Trial of a High n-3 Plus Low n-6 Diet." *Bipolar Disorders* 24, no. 2 (2022): 171–184. https://doi.org/10.1111/bdi.13112.

Sun, Jian-Long, Hong-Fang Ji, and Liang Shen. "Impact of Cooking on the Antioxidant Activity of Spice Turmeric." *Food Nutrition Research* 63 (2019): fnr.v63.3451. https://doi.org/10.29219/fnr.v63.3451.

Valls-Pedret, Cinta, Aleix Sala-Vila, Mercè Serra-Mir, Dolores Corella, Rafael de la Torre, Miguel Ángel Martínez-González, Elena H. Martínez-Lapiscina, Montserrat Fitó, Ana Pérez-Heras, Jordi Salas-Salvadó, et al. "Mediterranean Diet and Age-Related Cognitive Decline: A Randomized Clinical Trial." *Journal of the American Medical Association* 175, no. 7 (2015): 1094–1103. https://doi.org/10.1001/jamainternmed.2015.1668.

van Gelder, B.M., B. Buijsse, M. Tijhuis, S. Kalmijn, S. Giampaoli, A. Nissinen, and D. Kromhout. "Coffee Consumption Is Inversely Associated with Cognitive Decline in Elderly European Men: The FINE Study." *European Journal of Clinical Nutrition* 61 (2007): 226–232. https://doi.org/10.1038/sj.ejcn.1602495.

Zielinska, Magdalena, Edyta Łuszczki, Izabela Michońska, and Katarzyna Dereń. "The Mediterranean Diet and the Western Diet in Adolescent Depression—Current Reports." *Nutrients* 14, no. 20 (2022): 4390. https://doi.org/10.3390/nu14204390.

INDEX

Page references in *italics* indicate photographs

About the Authors

Serena Ball, MS, RD, and Deanna Segrave-Daly, RD, each have more than twenty years of culinary nutrition experience and have dedicated their careers to helping people make delicious and nutritious meals. Together, they are the authors of four Mediterranean diet cookbooks. Deanna lives in Philadelphia with her husband and daughter, and Serena lives outside St. Louis with her husband and five children. You can find them online at teaspoonofspice.com and doing weekly live-stream recipe demonstrations on their Facebook page, Teaspoon of Spice.

ACKNOWLEDGMENTS

A huge thank you to our exquisite editor Claire Schulz and awesome agent Clare Pelino, who made cookbook writing for us a possibility and a joy. Also a shout out to the ultra-talented Elise Cellucci, whose gorgeous photos take our recipes to the next level. We're grateful for the incredible team that backs us at BenBella Books, including Lindsay Marshall, Kim Broderick, Sarah Avinger, and Karen Wise. Appreciation and good luck to our dietetic intern Kevin McCall. And lastly, the biggest and most humble gratitude to our families, friends, recipe testers, and loyal followers—another cookbook dedicated to all of you!

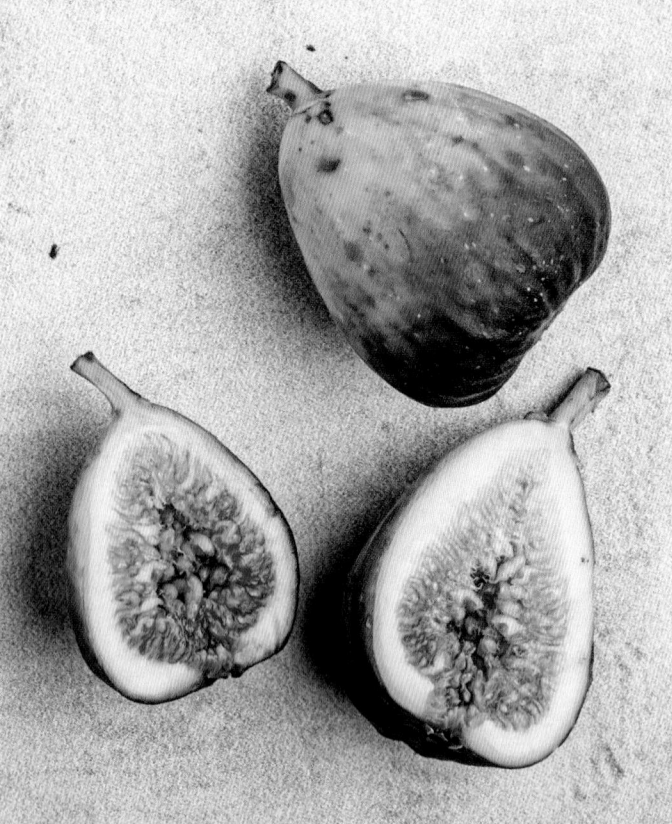